Jim's Hands
Hope
Mother-in-law

The picture on the front of the book was painted by my mother-in-law, Hope Lebo.

My wife and I took our vacation the week before football season in Florida to visit our mother. She had learned to paint and asked me if I wanted her to do one for me.

I said, "Would you paint my hands." I had so many operations that the medicine was taking the pigment out of my whole body and my hands were the worst.

Mom asked, "Why the hands?"

I answered, "See how bad my hands look, I want to share with those who come for a massage, that with hands as bad as mine, God can still use them."

Mom took a picture of my hands and did an oil painting of them, then sent the oil painting to us in a couple of weeks.

The oil painting was hung up in the waiting room of my Sport Therapy Center. I was asked about the painting and was pleased with the opportunity of sharing what the painting stood for.

I dedicate my story to
Our Children
Mary Louise Cockrell and Husband Bill Cockrell
Grandson Dain Alexander Cockrell
Robert James Byron and Wife Gina Byron
Step-grandson Dylan Finn
Our Mothers and Fathers
Brothers and Their Wives

Thanks to Terry Husky, friend and neighbor, who help me to edit my life's story.

Also thanks to Michael J. Garrett of Garrett Photography for layout, design and helping me get it published.

Copyright © 2011 by Jim Byron

All rights reserved except as permitted under the U.S. Copyright Act of 1976, no part of this publication may be reproduced, distributed, or transmitted in any form or by any means, or stored in a database or retrieval system, without the prior written permission of the publisher.

Front Cover photo Copyright © 2011 by Illa Byron

THE HEALING TOUCH

JIM BYRON

1

On March 21, 1931, the frigid western Pennsylvania morning held the promise of spring and the dire realization that the anniversary of this date might never be celebrated.

Dr. Winters held the newborn baby in his arms while talking to the mother. "Have you ever seen such a beautiful baby?"

"He's beautiful, all right," she said.

"Look how little he is, Anne." Dr. Winters placed the baby in his mother's arms.

"He's not very big, is he?" Anne said, gazing at her son.

Dr. Winters looked out the window. "You're fortunate to be in a warm room. It's cold outside." He turned back to her. "How are you doing?"

"I'm tired but I feel good."

"You should, after delivering a baby boy," he said.

"I'm okay. Still it seemed like a long day."

"Your delivery went smoothly."

"It was good that I didn't have to wait or work very long," she smiled.

"Are you in any pain?"

"No. I feel good for having delivered a baby."

"Were you able to rest?" he asked.

"Yes, I've had a good night's sleep. You know Dr. Winters, I appreciate your concern."

"Do you need anything?"

"No, I'm doing okay. Thank you for asking."

"Anne, I need to discuss something with you. There is a problem," he said gently.

"What kind of problem?" She looked at the doctor and frowned.

"Your son has a defect," he said very softly.

"What kind of defect?" she asked with fear in her eyes, as she stared at her doctor. She had known him for many years through the church and because he had delivered her other children.

"He has spina bifida," Dr. Winters said.

Her heart started to beat a little faster. "My younger sister has spina bifida. I was very young when she was born and I'm afraid I don't know much about it. I know my sister occasionally walks with a cane, but most of the time, she's in a wheelchair. Does this run in families?"

"Yes, it's hereditary. It's a congenital defect."

"What do you mean?" The crease in her forehead deepened as she rubbed her son's shoulders.

"It means present at birth," he said.

"What is it exactly?" her voice quivered.

"Your son has an open hole located in his back near his tail bone."

"What caused it?" she asked as her breathing became labored.

"It's caused by the closure of the spinal column with herniated protrusions of the meninges of the spinal cord."

"I'm afraid I don't understand." She stroked her son's hair.

"The spinal column is bulging out."

"Why and how did this happen?" Anne asked.

"It occurs when there is damage to the embryo during the first weeks of pregnancy. During the twenty-fourth or twenty-fifth day, the spinal column closes and seals the spine to protect it. It's probably due to a combination of genetic and environmental factors."

"I don't understand."

"If there is anything foreign in the spinal column, such as a sliver of bone or a hair particle, the antibodies will attack and the pressure will force an opening. The opening starts out small and will increase in size as it comes to the surface of the skin. It may be no bigger than a dimple, or it can be as wide as four or five inches."

"I still don't understand." Dr. Winters took time to explain more about the antibodies.

"If too much spinal fluid drains into the brain, it will enlarge the skull to two-thirds the size of the body. This is known as a hydrocephalic head."

"What effect will that have?" she asked, as she hugged her son.

"He won't be able to move."

"Why, what will stop him?"

"If he tries to sit up, the weight of his head would break his neck. He would be confined to his bed for the rest of his life."

Anne clutched her baby as her eyes widened with fear. "And if the fluid doesn't drain into the brain?"

"The other possibility is a micro cephalic head."

"You mean there's another problem?" she asked as her body shivered.

"Yes. The head could decrease in size because of the lack of spinal fluid flowing in the brain. Hydrocephalic and micro cephalic children do not have a very long life expectancy."

The fear in Anne's eyes increased as she learned about the horrors of her son's spina bifida.

"What can be done for my son?" she asked as her hands started to sweat.

"He must have surgery," he answered. "Generally, the child should be operated on within the first twenty-four hours."

"Why does he have to have the surgery so quickly?"

"Infection may occur because of the open hole. The operation must be done to close it, to protect him."

"When are you going to operate on him?" she asked.

Dr. Winters said, "I'm not going to operate on your son right away. I want to wait until the opening stops growing."

"Why would you wait, knowing my son could die without the operation?"

"If his operation is done too soon the antibodies attacking the skin may force a split in the sutures because of the opening expansion. Waiting until the hole reaches its full size provides a better chance for your son's survival. I want to do one surgery instead of two. He should survive one operation. I doubt that he'd survive two."

"How long before you do the surgery?"

"I'm not sure."

"You're saying my son doesn't have much chance for survival. Is that what you're saying?"

Dr. Winters hesitated, looked into her eyes and said, "Yes, Anne. This is a very difficult operation."

"How will you know when to operate? I don't want him to suffer."

"I'll look in on him every day."

"What if he has an infection?"

"If there is that possibility, he'll be operated on immediately."

"What other problems could he face?" Tears welled in her eyes. "I'm sorry, this is hard for me to grasp." She looked at her son. Her voice broke, "Will there be any other complications from the surgery?"

"The surgery is dangerous. He may not live through it."

"Why?" she asked while caressing her son.

"The nerves are intertwined like string in a baseball. I have to be very careful not to cut the spinal nerve. This will cause the lower extremities to be paralyzed from this delicate operation. The surgery could take a long time."

"How long will it take?"

"It could be anywhere from four to eight hours. My major concern is that your son's heart is strong enough to endure such a long surgery. It's important that I go slowly. I don't want to cut the spinal nerve. It will take time to separate the nerves. The surgery requires a lot of concentration and patience. I'll be able to see what must be done while closing the hole."

"Will he be paralyzed?"

"If the nerve to the lower extremities is cut, he will be."

"How soon will you know if he can move his legs?"

"He'll move his legs when he's stretching after the operation."

"How long can he be expected to live?"

"He'll live one to four years with surgery, less without it."

"You mean to tell me, my son will not live any longer than four years?" her voice shook.

"Yes Anne, that's the life expectancy of a spina bifida child. He may live until he's seven and a half years old. If he lives longer than that, he'll be mentally retarded. I'll do everything that's possible to keep him alive."

Dr. Winters picked up the baby and took him back to the nursery. He wanted her to hold the child while hearing what he had to say about the spina bifida.

Dr. Winters was a general practitioner who always listened to what was said. His outstanding characteristic was his love for his patients. Anne knew this because he gave her all the answers to her questions.

She was exhausted and stunned by the realization of what was ahead for her son. Anne thought about all the things Dr. Winters had told her. The pressure she felt was so heavy that it made it difficult for her to breathe.

She spent the time praying and asking God what she must do. Her faith was so strong; she felt God would provide the guidance in making the best decision for her son. She knew her son would be treated as if he were normal and be given the best service that the doctor could provide.

Her faith in God would make a difference. At that moment, it was difficult for her to see how anything could be changed. So much information and pressure made it difficult to focus on God and allow Him to touch her heart. She needed God to take away this terrible feeling of fear.

God had used the spina bifida to draw her closer to Him than ever before. She needed His understanding and direction to know what must be done to benefit her child. She knew that God would increase her faith by providing the answers that were needed. No matter how much she prayed, it was difficult for her to get rid of the desperation she felt in her heart.

"God give me the energy and strength to deal with whatever situation spina bifida causes," she prayed. "Help me to have a clear mind to make the right decisions that will add years to his life."

This lady was spiritually tough and walked with God daily. She shared everything with Him as good friends do. She was my mother. My name is Jim Byron. I was born with spina bifida and this is my story.

2

Dr. Winters operated on me when I was five and a half months old. It was a long hospital stay and he came in every day before the surgery to check for infection.

Dr. Winters thought someone should be in my room for the first twenty-four hours after the surgery. There weren't enough nurses for one to spend all night with one patient, so my Aunt Louise was sitting with me when Dr. Winters walked into my room.

"I think Jim moved his legs," Aunt Louise said.

"Oh, you want him to move his legs so badly that you probably just imagined it."

"I'm sure I saw them move."

Dr. Winters looked over Aunt Louise's shoulder and saw me lifting my legs and stretching. My movements eased his greatest fear and my chance of survival was good for now.

He was very happy with the outcome of the surgery but continued to warn my family that I'd probably not live to see my next birthday. The tests he ran supported this.

Dr. Winters said that even though the operation was a success, there might be some brain damage. He felt so strongly about this that he told my parents: "If Jimmy lives to be seven and a half years old, he will be mentally retarded." All the medical literature supported his statement.

Shortly after surgery, I left the hospital and back home I'd jabber one moment and blackout the next. This usually occurred in the morning during breakfast. When this happened, my parents would take me to the living room couch and put cold packs on my forehead. It was done so naturally and casually that my brothers were never alarmed. After these episodes my parents would call Dr. Winters to make sure I was okay.

The blackouts occurred between the ages of six months and two years with more frequency in the early months. The origin was never determined. It was extremely stressful and frustrating for my parents who were powerless to prevent my suffering.

This situation only deepened their dependence on the Lord. They trusted God to provide the strength to do whatever was needed. They knew without a doubt that He would take care of things.

When I was three years old, Dr. Winters referred my parents to a number of doctors in western Pennsylvania to try to find out if there was anything that could be done for my spina bifida. The test results indicated my life expectancy wasn't very long. Mom asked each doctor how our family could make a difference.

Whenever doctors suggested placing me in an institution, my parents refused. They asked a lot of questions about what could be done for me and how they could best care for me while I was alive. They understood the impossible odds they faced, the ninety percent mortality rate for spina bifida children in 1934. They didn't expect me to live long, but the family would provide whatever I needed. My mother told the doctors, "My son will have the support of our family. No matter what happens, we'll lean on the Lord for direction. God will provide what we need. Jim will know that we are there for him and will understand that he's not going through any difficult problems alone. We will enjoy him as long as he lives and he will be treated as if he were normal."

When I left the hospital, Mom was in a black mood because of the possibility of my death. Dad tried teasing Mom to cheer her up while driving home.

I was standing on the floor, behind the front seat, on the driver's side. I put my arms around Dad's neck and said after one of his funny remarks, "Dad, the only thing funny about you is your face." They both laughed and it helped to break the tension.

My parents said nothing about the doctors' comments and it was hard for me to understand why they were so sad. It was important for them to remain cheerful and not give me any cause for worry, though I wasn't smart enough to worry about it anyway.

Mom and Dad felt it was a waste of time to worry about things they couldn't change. They were too busy looking for ways to make a difference in my life.

Their concentration on finding solutions did not permit self-pity to reside in their hearts and heads. Their concern was my spina bifida. Mom and Dad believed every situation we faced came from God. The good ones provided a spiritual blessing that uplifted our hearts and gave us the desire to follow God's lead. They also believed God allowed difficult situations to come into our lives so we could develop a spiritual toughness and a strong faith. My parents stayed in communication with God and they always prayed for guidance. I could see, by their walk with God, that there was no doubt He was by their side. This relationship uplifted their hearts and provided the wisdom to deal with each difficult problem with a happy spirit.

My parents were strong Christians. Their faith was so strong that they believed God would take them home to Heaven when they died. God was their friend with whom they could and did share everything from their heart. Each of us took a turn leading the prayer before each meal, which began after everyone was seated.

Mom and Dad believed church was so important that we were expected to attend Church and Sunday school as well as Wednesday night prayer meetings. The standard rule was if you were too sick to go to Sunday school, then you were too sick to go out and play after church. This was rarely an issue since we all enjoyed going to church and didn't want to miss.

The most outstanding characteristic in our family was the love shown to all six boys. Each one of us thought we were the favorite. We were taught to love and respect each other and we followed our parents' example, leaning on the Lord whenever we had a problem.

Mom took me to see Dr. Winters for two shots a day from April until late September. Without these shots seizures or infections might have ended my life.

When it was time for my shots, I'd run off to hide and Mom had to send my brothers to find me. It didn't matter where I hid; someone always found me and brought me home to Mom for a good scolding. I shouldn't say a "good scolding," because none of it was ever "good." She always explained how important these shots were and missing them could be life-threatening. I didn't know what "life-threatening" was, but Mom was so serious, I knew it must be bad.

We spent most of our time each day waiting for Dr. Winters to give me the shots. As soon as I walked into his office, he'd ask, "How are you doing, Jimmy?" And then follow up with, "Are you ready for your shots?"

Those shots terrified me, but I acted tough by talking out the side of my mouth like a gangster. I asked, "Whatta ya mean, am I ready? I just walked in here. You're not gonna give me a shot." Both of us knew it was coming. Dr. Winters wasn't fooled by my tough act.

After a while, he said, "Come on Jimmy, it's time for your shots."

I really thought my actions fooled him, but this beautiful gentle doctor knew my tough act was used to hide my fear of the shots.

I'd muster up my toughest voice and say in a loud deep voice, "Okay Doc, let's get it over with."

He gave me the shots and asked, "Now Jimmy, that didn't hurt did it?"

My answer always made him smile. "You're right Doc, it didn't hurt you at all because you gave me the shots." I loved Dr. Winters and did whatever he said needed to be done. His love allowed me enough time to prepare myself for anything. He allowed a tough-minded kid to have his act. How could you not love a doctor as special as he was?

Dr. Winters told my mother, "Jimmy makes my day. He acts so tough but still will do whatever I ask him. He's a special little guy. I have many patients who come to see me who are not really sick. If they had Jimmy's beautiful spirit, they would be too busy to take the time to see me."

I learned it's okay to say, I'm hurting, but not to make a big deal out of it and not to dwell on my problems. So I was born with spina bifida and I had to learn to live with it. That sounds harsh, but I needed that attitude to deal with the severe pain as well as the other problems that go with the disability.

My family was always there during the toughest times. I never went through the severe pain by myself. They felt the same pain I did. God gave us the strength to face anything. His spirit made a difference because He was in the middle of whatever occurred in our family.

Dad was a well-respected man in our community. His day started early in the morning and continued late at night. He worked long hours to make his grocery store successful. Dad also enjoyed what he was doing, especially taking care of his customers. He had a great sense of humor and customers enjoyed being around him. No one wanted to leave because they were having so much fun.

He treated everyone the way he wanted to be treated, with love and understanding. He didn't have to say a word; his actions spoke volumes about Christ's love. This was the best way to witness to those who came into his store.

My dad used jokes around the house because he didn't want to frighten my brothers and have them worry about the severity of my condition. Once while I was jabbering away in my highchair, I suddenly went into a seizure. Dad made jokes and had everyone laughing as he picked me up out of the highchair and took me into another room where he applied cold packs to my head until the doctor came.

Dad was an inspiration to all of us and our love for him was very strong. He always let us know how important we were to the family, especially me. Dad filled us with laughter and we received his undivided attention whenever we talked to him.

Whenever I had problems, no matter how trivial, he never seemed to mind. Many times he laughed at how I expressed what bothered me and helped me do what should be done.

3

On a hot muggy day when I was five years old, I went down to watch some friends wade in the creek three blocks from my home. The water came down from the hills and was so cold it felt good on the feet. Mom didn't allow me to wade in the creek because of the broken bottles. This was a place for target practice. Anyone who had a bottle threw it into the creek and then threw stones at the bottle trying to break it.

Sewage from nearby homes draining into the creek was another reason not to wade there. If anyone stepped on a broken bottle there was the possibility of infection, so most kids were very careful about where they stepped.

The kids continued to torment me about not wading with them. It was important for me to wade in the creek to prove I wasn't chicken. They knew that after a while I'd give in. The teasing intensified until I'd had enough. Finally my shoes and socks came off and I waded in the creek.

Everyone was playing around and not paying any attention to where they were stepping. I stepped on a broken milk bottle, cutting my foot across the arch and up under my toes. My foot was numb so I didn't realize it was cut until I saw blood in the water.

My foot really throbbed as I was coming out of the creek. I stepped on a stone that penetrated the deepest part of the cut. The pain was so severe that I yelled and the kids carried me home. As soon as I came into the house, Mom saw my foot and called Dr. Winters. Mom was upset but she didn't want me to suffer, even if I had disobeyed her. She felt the severe cut was enough punishment. Pleasing the kids instead of Mom taught me a hard lesson. If they wanted to call me chicken, that was okay. From then on, Mom's word was law. I'd listen to her.

My foot had to be elevated and there could be very little movement. When the kids were playing in our back yard, it was so hard to sit still and not go and join them. The severe cut prevented me from doing anything with them. The cut took a long time to heal because my foot was injured to the bone. My poor circulation prevented the blood flow that a normal foot would have. Trying to put weight on it caused more severe pain, like pouring salt on a cut. The burning sensation made it impossible for me to find a comfortable position for my foot. When finally the bandages were removed, Dr. Winters allowed me to walk on it. His suggestion was much easier said than done. When I took a step, the weight of my body applied so much pressure that the burning sensation intensified. It felt like sand was under my skin and the irritation rubbed my foot raw.

Despite the pain it was up to me to start walking. It took a while for me to build up the courage to step down on the ground, but each time it became easier.

The pain lingered after I lifted my foot off the ground and slowly I felt relief. That's why it took so long to attempt another step. I didn't want to face the pain. It made me a coward. Finally my desire to walk took over and I'd take a deep breath and start over. The pain was good for me because it taught me to endure and learn to adjust.

I'd never be intimidated by the kids' remarks, even though their teasing was difficult to ignore. My interest was not pleasing the kids; it was doing what Mom said and pleasing myself. If the kids didn't like it and called me chicken, it didn't matter. Any time something was asked of me, I'd look at the overall picture before trying something that could hurt me.

I'll never forget the severe pain. I remember every detail as if it were yesterday. The cut deformed my foot and caused pain for many years. Some lessons are hard to learn, but this one was good for me.

After the incident the kids feared I'd squeal on them, telling Mom they dared me to go into the creek. The kids were surprised that they weren't blamed. I was learning to be responsible for my actions. A person has to pay for what he does wrong. My price was a severely cut and deformed foot. The doctor had to stretch the skin to stitch it together. This caused my right foot to be a half size smaller than my left.

My foot had healed after cutting it in the creek, but the muscles were still very tender and extremely sensitive to touch. I'd put my shoe on my right foot as gently as possible. I'd unlace the shoe and spread it as wide as possible. If the toes on my right foot were slightly bumped it caused a bruise and my foot throbbed severely all day. The pain in my right foot made it too tender to walk. Despite the pain, walking was necessary and it was up to me to learn to live with it. The burning sensation never stopped. The heavy steel shank made the shoes impossible to put on without bumping my toes.

My feet were not only inverted, my right leg was two and a half inches shorter than my left. Dr. Winters had the idea of building the right shoe up two and a quarter inches. He thought the heavy weight of the shoe would stretch my leg to make it even with the other foot. Being a quarter inch shorter would cause my right foot to drop.

My mother took me to the shoe repairman to see if this idea was possible. He said he could do it and built up the right shoe to the specifications Dr. Winters wanted.

The weight of the heavy right shoe stretched my right leg. At first, the weight of the shoe didn't make much difference, but gradually my right foot started to drop a little. The pain from my hip down to my toes continued until the shoe reached the next quarter inch. The pain began as the spasm released and my leg dropped. Once the spasm released, the pain lessened and my leg became stronger. The pain decreased with each adjustment until my hips were not locked and I could move my feet forward.

My back hurt less as my right foot was able to carry more weight. A bone stuck out of the middle and side of my right foot and continually wore a hole in the side of my shoe which the shoemaker repeatedly patched. I didn't have enough strength to carry my right foot forward compared to my left foot. When walking, I'd whip my right foot around in a half circle. This applied pressure on the leather and caused the patch to wear out quickly. With regular repairs, I was able to wear the shoe for a couple of years until there was a sixteenth inch difference in my legs.

In response to the pain I complained, experienced frustration, and felt contempt for others. My family did everything possible to make my life easier and no one knew that as well as I did. If my moody behavior was out of hand, my parents addressed it by having me spend time alone in my room.

Having a family with strong spiritual love provided growth in my life. The severe physical pain made me angry and anger prevented me from moving away from the pain. My ability to deal with it developed slowly. It was difficult for me to see anything but the effect pain had on me. This attitude made me so hard to love and yet my family never failed to reach out and lift my spirit when I needed it most. My moods were devastating and I found it impossible to see God's light through my tunnel of depression. I thought someone had stolen the light bulb because my heart was pitch-black. I didn't allow God's love to shine through. It took a while but eventually God's love did shine through and enabled me to stop complaining.

My brother Tug had carried me wherever I wanted to go while I was wearing the casts. Despite the pressure of the responsibility to carry me from one place to another, he never complained that it was too much. Learning to walk with these shoes gave me the freedom to get up and go anywhere without having to depend on someone having to carry me.

Walking was an exciting freedom and a wheelchair would have deprived me of this opportunity. The pain continued to be a negative force and it sometimes hampered my desire to become more active. Exercise also strengthens the body so it was great for health reasons. The intense pain was more evident in the beginning, but after a while walking made it less severe.

Since spina bifida children weren't able to walk for very long, I thought it would be great to do what others hadn't done, but that was not my goal. Freedom of movement was the driving force.

4

My clothes were always wet and the strong urine smell was one of the reasons the kids I played with didn't want me near them. I didn't want to smell bad, so I would change whenever I lost control. I'd wash myself and put on clean clothes a number of times during the day, but still my clothes were wet.

Bladder control was so difficult that the continual effort was exhausting. I worked on it for a long time without any positive results. I held my stomach muscles in to give me more control, but the muscles were weak. It was impossible for me to hold the position for long and the effort tired me. As soon as my stomach muscles relaxed, I'd void without knowing it. Sometimes this occurred when I was talking with someone. I didn't know that my bladder had released until I felt the urine going down my leg. This was very embarrassing. It happened so often and the person I was talking to could see my wet clothes before I realized what had happened.

I was allowed to leave my yard as long as I was close enough to home to hear when my parents called me. I spent most of the time playing in my yard. Some of the kids who I thought were my friends ridiculed me severely. There were always four or five older kids making ugly comments. One started it by saying, "Do you still wet your pants, little baby?" and the rest joined in. Each comment was more painful than the last. The urine smell was so strong that my playmates smelled me long before I came into view. They resented the smell and seeing my wet clothes. They would say, "Is the little baby ever going to grow up? Do you still wear diapers?" The put-downs were fierce. I went home too embarrassed to say anything. No matter what I said or did the insults continued.

The most difficult problem was losing people I thought were my friends. As soon as I heard the comments I'd turn around and head for home. The kids yelled, "Why don't you stay and fight? Are you chicken?" As I ran for home, I looked over my shoulder making sure I wasn't being chased. I saw the kids mocking me and heard them making the sounds of a chicken in flight.

Sometimes I would tell Mom what they said and how they made fun of me.

"Do you say anything to them?" she asked.

"No. If I did, the kids would gang up on me. I can't lick four or five kids at one time. I don't want to fight because I'll lose what friends I have."

"But you have lots of friends," she said. "Kids come here to play with you all the time."

"They come over to play with my toys and pay no attention to me when I talk to them," I told Mom. "They'll look at me and say nothing."

I played with only one person at a time in our yard. My problem started when another playmate came into the yard. Then it was two against one. I would tell them to leave and pick up my toys and go into the house.

My mother would say, "If you boys can't be nice to Jimmy, don't come back." They would mock me as they left.

After that, I would go off by myself until my hot temper cooled down. I thought about what could be done. If what I did could be changed, I'd work on it. If it was something that I had no control over I'd try to forget and learn to live with it. My anger made it difficult for love to live in my heart instead of hate. I'd work on my feelings until the hate left my heart. The only way to do this was to keep my mind busy.

My problem with bladder control taught me many lessons. It taught me not to worry about something I could not control. I learned at an early age that regardless of the situation, you had to deal with problems head-on. Never be afraid to search for an answer you need to improve your life. The frustration of the physical pain and especially the ridicule provided a determination to make this bad situation work for me. Even when this didn't happen, I still made an effort to be as successful as I could.

My major challenge was turning this problem around to help me become a better person. I didn't want to be intimidated by anyone's comments. Even though it made me feel bad, I wasn't going to allow their actions to dictate my behavior. This was very hard to do.

Contempt filled my heart with hate instead of love. It was difficult to face those kids because the ridicule was so severe and unrelenting. My feelings were hurt and the embarrassment was so devastating that I didn't want to see them ever. I didn't do anything to bring on this thoughtless treatment. My heart was bitter and anger came to the surface after I left the kids. This made me unlovable. I was so hot that if anyone touched me, they'd have burned their hands. I'd go home and tell my mother what was said. She always listened and encouraged me and told me to ignore their comments, adding, "Jimmy, you have to rise above it." It took a long time, but my mother's love helped me to turn it around.

Contempt and ridicule were the most difficult areas for me to deal with. The devastation from the ridicule sometimes lasted more than a day. Their contempt broke my heart and caused me to wonder, "Will I ever find a place where someone will accept or even love me?"

The worthless feeling took away any positive thinking that God could help me. My thoughts were on self, not on how God could improve my attitude. Insecurity plagued me and I thought the kids would never accept me. They couldn't see past my spina bifida and sensed my vulnerability and used it against me. Their prejudice caused such negative feelings and I found it difficult to rise above it. The mental pain was so strong that my heart had a tough time adjusting. When my heart lost its desire to fight, the possibility of failure increased. Sometimes the mental and physical pain was too much to overcome.

The heart is the center of our spirit. If the heart is beaten and you feel the devastation, this will kill the spirit. God controlled my heart and anyone who ridiculed another, for any reason, was destroying God's gift of life. Whenever this happened to me I thought, "You're not going to get away with this. Do you think you can destroy me? I've got news for you, you'll never beat me." My spirit did not give up.

My disability required tremendous heart, just to deal with the physical pain. The ridicule placed more pressure on my heart to emotionally survive. If I did not persevere my life would not be successful. The struggle, regardless of how tough it was, enabled me to stay positive for God to have something to work with.

My concentration was on making the adjustment. It was important for me to always try to do my best. Gradually my anger left and God instilled a stronger determination to succeed no matter how many times I failed.

God was the only friend I had outside of my family. His love gave me an opportunity to stay on top even when losing. There was no doubt in my mind that anger would lead to failure. God pointed out that anger was my major problem most of the time. He gave me a positive outlook and made my life better, using the pain of the disability and prejudice to develop a spiritual toughness.

I was still angry when those who made the comments came toward me. In the beginning, I'd go the opposite way to avoid them. They had said, "I don't want to be around someone who smells as bad as you do." I didn't want to be around them either. Even when I was clean and didn't smell I'd still go my own way and stay away from their nasty comments because of the negative feeling it left in my heart.

I'd stay away from the kids until God had cleared my mind and heart of the hate that was living there. It took God a little longer because of my aggressive attitude in wanting to fight back. He had patience with me because of His love. With a positive attitude love lived in my heart instead of hate.

Now it was time to face the kids and show them what God had done for me. Whenever the kids saw me coming toward them, they couldn't understand why I didn't treat them the way I was treated. I knew from their sarcastic comments that their intent was to hurt my feelings. They didn't care about me they just wanted to see my reaction. They wanted to make me angry, but they weren't going to dictate how I felt. It happened so many times and I learned not to show my anger and not allow them to control my behavior.

When comments were made, I'd get up and leave as soon as it started. If I stayed, my playmates would form a circle around me so I couldn't get away.

Finally, my mother decided it was time for me to wear diapers. This went a long way in getting rid of the smell. My clothes were no longer wet and the comments about how bad I smelled stopped. I was going into first grade and it was time for me to get used to wearing something that gave a little more protection while going to school.

5

The kids in McGrann attended Bellwood School and I was looking forward to my first day of school. Mom was actually taking me to a place other than a hospital. This was exciting because school was a more inviting place. My legs were going as fast as my little body allowed. I thought if I didn't hurry someone might say it was time for me to return to the hospital. Anything had to be better than spending my time there.

Mom seemed to enjoy walking me to school. As we approached the building, most of the kids were looking out the window at me. They may have seen me as a crippled kid coming down the street heading for school, but it was still a happy day for me. Can you imagine what a thrill it was to go to school? Boy that was special.

In the beginning of the school year, the kids were kind to me. They brought me into the game as a referee in order to include me as much as possible. Gradually, this kindness wore off and the ridicule started. One day it was how I looked and walked. It didn't matter, if there was something they could make fun of, I would hear about it. I knew if I said anything, their comments would get worse.

Life up to this point was very difficult. School was another area that moved my frustration up a couple of notches. The teacher knew I had trouble understanding what she said. I asked so many questions and still didn't understand. My learning didn't progress much and I was considered slow. Many of my teachers believed my failure was the result of not listening to what was said or read. "Did you hear what I said?" they would say.

"I heard you but I don't understand."

"You'll have to pay attention and listen."

My teachers didn't do much to help me to understand. It was normal for me to fail. After a long, long time my failure turned into success because of my continual effort to succeed. I was able to understand the lesson.

Then all of a sudden without any warning, I'd be rushed to the hospital. I'd spend time at home recuperating until I was well enough to return to school. I missed a lot of school and when I returned, the teacher was so far ahead on the new subject that I was never able to catch up. This added to my frustration.

My teacher's comments about my being a slow learner only intensified my desire to learn. As a result of this and with my mother's help, I was able to develop good study habits. My grades didn't improve quickly, but I was gradually learning even though the progress was slow.

Somehow my physical disability inspired me to be successful. If my goal could not be attained one way, I'd look for a different route. Each failure strengthened my determination to work harder. It would come; I just had to be patient. Failure was no excuse for not trying. Learning was tough because of my inability to concentrate on what was said. No matter how many times I failed, my mother's faith in me didn't allow me to quit.

It was a long hard process but when I finally learned the assignment I never forgot the information. Mom spent hours going over the material with me until it was second nature to me. Whenever a particular part of the assignment was very difficult, I'd make up a funny story to remember it. The process worked for me and Mom enjoyed my stories.

The spina bifida caused many bladder infections and severe physical pain. I was hospitalized many times and in and out of school for the next three years.

At the end of the school year the teacher promoted students to the next grade. My attendance was below the number of days you had to be in school to pass. As a result, I flunked first grade twice. The kids took advantage of my failures to make sure I knew how dumb I was. I always thought my failing was because I did not learn as much as was expected. I didn't find out until years later that if I had stayed in school the required days, I would have been promoted to the next grade.

The kids made sarcastic comments about how funny I walked. This made me feel worthless and crushed my spirit. My feet were still inverted to the center of my body which caused poor balance. The unusual gait made me look awkward. My long arms and short body made the kids think I walked like a monkey. This wasn't so bad to deal with, but the sarcastic laughter was.

The anger built up resentment toward the kids, making the pressure feel like it would blow my head off my shoulders. My heart was broken. I didn't see how God could ever put the pieces back together again and give me a positive attitude.

Whenever I would get angry at what the kids had said, I'd go off by myself and talk with God. It was important to tell Mom where I was. The possibility that I'd black out or have a seizure caused my mother a lot of concern. If I were missing for a long time, she would know where to look for me. Once alone I'd pour out my hate and pain to God.

"Will anyone ever love me? Am I so bad that people hate me so much? Will I ever be treated with kindness? If so, when and where will it happen?" These thoughts brought hot stinging tears to my eyes.

As I sat there with my head bowed, my body shaking racked with pain from the ridicule, I couldn't stop crying. God filled my heart with a gentle warmth that soothed my body. There was a powerful love so soft and warm, that it took away my anger. Each time this happened the Lord helped me develop an inner toughness. God provided a feeling of love that enabled me to believe in myself, strong enough to handle anything. God was always there for me and He always let me know I wasn't alone.

My self-pity was so severe that I felt God was the only one who could cleanse my heart of this devastating feeling. He always touched my heart in a special way. His love took away the self-pity and helped me to focus on the hate that caused my bad attitude. When I finally faced the problem and dealt with it, God took away the sting and replaced it with His love. This enabled me to forgive the kids for what they had said.

I felt God had made me special. Regardless of what happened to me, no one was going to destroy the gift God gave me. My physical disability was the part of His plan for me.

If you have heart, you cannot be beaten, but prejudice, ridicule and contempt can threaten spiritual survival. My disability required tremendous heart, just to deal with the physical pain, but the ridicule placed more pressure on my heart to emotionally survive. If this were allowed, I would never be successful. The struggle, regardless of how tough it was, enabled me to stay positive and give God something to work with.

It was important for me to always try to do my best. Gradually my anger would leave and God instilled a stronger determination to succeed no matter how many times I failed. His love gave me the opportunity to stay on top even when losing. There was no doubt in my mind that anger caused my failure. God pointed out that anger was my major problem most of the time. He gave me a positive outlook and made my life better, using the pain of the disability and ridicule to test me.

6

When I was in the first grade, I would often go to the junkyard after school to play. I'd stand in an old wrecked car pretending to be one of the racecar drivers on a dirt track. Racing was a very popular sport in western Pennsylvania and it was a lot of fun for many of the young people at that time. Like the rest of the kids, I sped down my mind's track and headed for the junkyard to pretend I was racing.

Most of the time if my brother Shun wasn't around, I'd play by myself because no one wanted to play with me. My mind was active and I'd come up with some of the craziest situations to entertain myself.

I had just walked across the street from the junkyard and was about three blocks from home when Ron and some of his friends saw me. It was about five o'clock and I was heading home for supper. One of Ron's friends yelled, "There's Jim, let's get him!" As soon as I heard that, I ran for home. It didn't take Ron and his gang long to catch up with me. While chasing me they mocked and made fun of how bad I looked. This was going to be a bad evening.

I was surprised they paid any attention to me. Ron and his friends were a couple years older and had never bothered me. Now they bumped and pushed, trying to knock me down. I ran about two and a half blocks. The running exhausted me and jarred my body with increasing pain from head to toe.

If I ran too fast, my right foot would rotate, hit the back of my left knee, and cause me to fall. Finally, one of Ron's friends poked a stick between my knees and I was on the ground.

While lying there, the kids hit me with sticks and stones. I protected my face and especially my eyes from being hit.

There was a long steel bolt about a foot long, lying next to me on the ground. When the kids weren't watching me, I'd stretch a little, gradually reaching for the bolt. No one paid any attention to this. They were too busy making fun of my size and looks. I reached out and grabbed the bolt and threw it into the crowd of kids. That stopped them.

I thought these kids needed to know what it felt like to be on the receiving end of some punishment. Given a chance to provide that punishment, I'd do it. My heart was full of hate and the bolt evened the odds.

The kids stood around the person I hit to see how bad it was. I stood for a moment without moving. I took a couple of steps, waiting for the ambush; still no one paid any attention to me. That's when I ran as fast as I could. It didn't take me long to get out of there. I stayed out of the house until about 9:00 P.M. That was my bedtime, and I knew being late would only mean more trouble.

When I walked into the house, Mom was waiting for me and said, "Uncle Dunc was here and said you hit Ron with a bolt. Did you hit him?"

"I knew someone was hit, but I didn't know who. Those kids were hitting me with sticks and stones, laughing and calling me names."

"You hit Ron above the eyelid. You could have put his eye out!" She was really angry and screamed, "Do you know that?" I'd never seen Mom so angry.

"No Mom, I didn't know Ron was the one I hit. All that was important to me was to get out of there and for the kids to stop picking on me."

"Ron had twelve stitches above his eye," she said.

"Mom, I don't like to fight but Ron had it coming. I'll do it again to stop them from picking on me. Maybe it did some good and he learned something because I surely did. No matter how I defend myself, I'm wrong and Ron is always right. Well, he better not mess with me again."

Mom sat there and didn't say anything so there wasn't any reason for me to stick around. It was better for me to leave because it was evident that Mom was not only angry with me, her anger indicated she didn't love me anymore. I needed to leave Mom and go off by myself to work this out.

I left the house with a heavy broken heart. I felt Mom didn't love me, so why should I tell her where I was going? After an incident like this, my heart was filled with hate. Not only did the kids hate me, but also in defending myself, my anger let Mom down. Her disappointment was difficult to deal with because she had never been that angry with me.

My thoughts plagued me. How in the world, will I ever have a mother who'll love me again? What can be done to change Mom's feeling toward me? How could I do such a thing to her? If Mom didn't support me anymore, my loss would be devastating.

Again, I talked with God. Walking toward a quiet place, I prayed, "God, do You really know what it is like not to have a mother to love You?"

How could I face God and share my feelings when my heartbreak was so severe? It was impossible for me to feel love from anyone, if I felt that bad. How could God love someone as bad as me? There was so much hate in my heart.

How could I share my feelings when the shame made me feel so worthless? This was the worst day of my life. Never before had my heart hurt so much.

The feeling of rejection had such a devastating effect. Finally, after reaching a quiet solitary place, I let my heart go. I talked to God and shared my feelings with Him. My heart broke and tears rolled down over my cheeks like an open faucet. My shoulders shook violently because the sting of losing Mom's love was too much to bear. All my frustration was poured out to God, telling Him what I'd done, the kids' reactions and finally how Mom reacted. This last part was hard to admit, that Mom didn't love me anymore. It was the first time in my life I felt defeated.

I sat by myself not saying anything, trying to calm down. Knowing from experience that to deal with this problem, I would have to bring my attitude to a place where my problems could be recognized. Only then could God touch my heart. My attitude was not good and it required a lot of love to turn it around. Only God could do that.

It took quite a while, but God was able to touch my spirit with His gentle love. I prayed, "What can I do to make Mom see the change in me and love me again? Why did I do such a thing to her? How can I get over this terrible feeling?"

To this day, I don't know of a more difficult time in my life. With all this damage done I had to find a way to repair it. I had to restore my relationship with Mom.

Thoughts continued to pour through my mind. Doesn't anyone know how hard it is to take this abuse without fighting back, or understand the pain in my body and know how hard it is to live in here? Does anyone really care how I feel? Will it always be like this? If I defend myself will I always be wrong?

I wasn't able to see myself as a nice person. Gradually God's love entered my heart and gently took away the devastating sting of pain. It was only then my spirit was ready to return.

After a long time, I went back home. At this point, with feelings that Mom did not love me anymore, I didn't know if I had a home. Mom was there and told me how disappointed she was. "Mom, what would you have done in my place?" I asked. "You have a group of kids standing over you and they're hitting you with sticks and stones. Are you going to stay there and take it? You may be able to do that, but I can't. Do you really know what it feels like to be hated the way these kids hate me?" Mom saw my frustration and told me, as she had so many times, "Jimmy, you've got to rise above it and walk away."

"Mom, sometimes I'm not able to do that." At this point, feeling no support from Mom, my heart broke again. The tears rolled off my face and down my cheeks.

"Jimmy, I love you. I know you're having a rough time and I understand." That was what I needed to hear. I realized then, even though Mom was disappointed, she still loved me. Mom's love was my richest blessing and I resolved never to disappoint her again.

7

The kids saw me many times after that, but didn't try to intimidate me. Ron and his friends just ignored me. It was a great feeling to be left alone and not have to defend myself.

Ron's father came into my father's grocery store one day while I was reading some new comic books. Dad knew that I was sitting behind the counter. The comic books were on a bookshelf that stood about five feet tall. I couldn't be seen unless you went around the corner and stood in front of the bookcase.

As soon as I heard his voice, it didn't take me long to scoot up to the opposite corner of the bookcase. Thinking he'd come around and see me, I crawled into the opening on the other side, hidden from sight. I waited a long time before leaving the store. To my surprise, he was standing on the top step talking to a neighbor.

Ron's father saw me and said, "Jimmy, I want to talk to you." The neighbor left and he said, "Why did you hit Ron with the bolt? You could have put his eye out."

"Yes sir, you're right. I could have done that. The reason for throwing the bolt was to stop Ron and the kids from hitting me with sticks and stones."

"Ron said he didn't do anything to you."

"If Ron said that, he's lying to you."

"You can't be hitting people with bolts."

"What would you have done if you had a bunch of kids beating on you?"

"You still shouldn't be hitting on anyone."

I was very angry and said, "It's all right for Ron to do the hitting, but it isn't for anyone else! I'll tell you this, if Ron ever does that to me again, he'll get more of the same. If you want to protect him, then keep him away from me. You're only interested in what I've done. You haven't heard a word I've said. Whether you want to believe it or not, Ron was wrong for picking on me. I was wrong for hitting him with the bolt. I know that, but you can't allow him to go around picking on kids who can't defend themselves."

Ron's father didn't say any more to me. He turned and left. It seemed this problem wasn't ever going to end. My spirits were very low. My feelings were hurt because, no matter what was said, I was always wrong. Ron's father was disgusted by my actions and lack of remorse and his treatment of me made me feel worthless.

After talking to Ron's father, I went back into the store. Dad was standing at the counter and heard everything that was said. He appreciated the fact that my actions were not disrespectful to Ron's father.

Dad in his quiet way let me know I was still special in his eyes. He was there for me and I knew by the expression on his face that he really loved me.

Wow! What an awesome feeling that was. At least he never made me feel worthless. Do you know what a beautiful feeling that is, to have your dad there, supporting you, when no one else does? It seemed every time I experienced a feeling of worthlessness, God sent someone to love me and change that feeling to one of love. Dad had done that for me. No wonder he was the kind of person I wanted to be when I grew up someday. He was always there for me.

8

My parents taught me that God was my strength. He would provide whatever I needed. This gave me the strength to rise above my problems. My concentration was too busy fighting the pain. There wasn't time to blame anyone. My energy was needed to take care of the problems at hand. It was important never to ask for something that was impossible to change.

In the beginning, my griping caused most of the ridicule. This made me aggressive and difficult to be around. Even when people said things that were not unkind, it was hard for me to see the difference. The community had a hard time looking past my grumbling. My disability was not the reason for my rejection. People were just reacting to my aggressive behavior.

My physical disability wasn't very nice to see and I thought the community wanted me out of sight, or locked up in a closet so no one would see me. It was hard to fight the prejudice. The only support came from my family. My stubborn attitude did not allow me to accept this type of treatment from the community. This caused me to gripe a lot, which was a major reason for their feelings. I was determined to prove them wrong by not complaining.

Once my heart changed acceptance began. The community, to their surprise, saw a struggling young boy working very hard to deal with his pain. They saw the tenacity of my strength, and how these adverse comments fueled my desire to succeed.

I didn't want to fight. Fighting could mean the loss of a friend and I had very few. I'd only fight if someone else started it. I would defend myself only when there was no way out of a fight.

No one noticed any change in my aggressive attitude in the beginning because my temper would still explode once in a while. Gradually working on my bad attitude, I began to control my anger much better. People started to take notice of my improved attitude and saw a difference in me.

The love of my family and how closely my parents walked with God made a tremendous difference in my life. My parents, Aunt Louise, and my brothers were always there for me, even when my attitude was unlovable. Their love and support turned stumbling blocks into stepping stones.

Other people angered me and their attitudes were difficult to overcome. The belief that, "since he's a cripple, he's not smart enough to recognize ridicule. He doesn't know any better, so we can say anything about him. He won't understand." That kind of remark is like throwing mud against a wall, it may not stick, but it will leave a mark. This was insulting and made me more determined to change their attitude, even if it meant being in a fighting mood. I would stand and say, "I do understand what you're saying and you better not say it again." This was so devastating and my bitterness overwhelmed me. It was impossible for me to shake the feeling of worthlessness. It took a long time to recover from the ridicule.

Again I'd go off by myself and share my feelings with God. With a heart full of bitterness I would ask, "How will I ever face those people again?"

God gradually touched my heart with His love and my bitterness left. When the pressure of bitterness was released, it opened up a way for God's love to come into my heart. It was so important to find a solution because the mental pain left such negative feelings. My life needed positive reinforcement from God. I forgave the kids who wronged me and had no ill feelings in my heart toward them. Treating them with respect came from God because I was fighting mad and wanted to crack some heads together. To the kids' surprise I was kind to them. God replaced my anger with a renewed love that lifted my spirit.

9

In my opinion, the closeness and stability of our family seemed to be the exception in our community. My brothers would argue as brothers do, but they always respected each other. I always considered Christ a family member. Because of our faith in Him, He was involved in whatever we did. Even though our family was struggling through the Depression, Christ's love was the major reason for our family's happiness and fulfillment.

My parents' struggle really made an impression on my life. As important as money was to keep us alive, our treatment of each other was more important. This was what our parents instilled in our lives.

During the Depression, many families had no money for food. Dad gave them credit for their groceries even though he knew many of them would never be able to pay him back. His heart was too big to turn them away. Many years later, some who couldn't afford to pay during the Depression became well-to-do, but never offered to pay our family what they owed.

The pressure of the Depression and trying to make ends meet was very difficult for my Dad. My problems with spina bifida and doctors' warnings that I wouldn't live very long caused Dad to have stomach ulcers. At first, it was stomach cramps and the pain gradually worsened. Dad went to Dr. Winters and talked to him about the pain. He advised Dad to have an operation to remove the ulcer. The surgery was successful and Mom went to see him after the operation. Dad was resting comfortably and told Mom, "If anything happens to me and I don't come through this, I'll see you in Heaven."

After the visit Mom went home. She didn't want to tire him. Mom rode the bus about five miles to our home. She had just walked into the house when the phone rang. Dad had become very ill. She was asked to come to the hospital as quickly as possible, because Dad might not make it. Mom was there to see Dad a few minutes before he died. Dad had gone into shock and there wasn't any medicine at that time to stabilize him.

Mom came into our bedroom to see my brother Shun and me. Even though I was only seven and a half, I was the older brother. Shun was five. "I want to talk to both of you." We could see that she was upset and very sad.

Shun and I got up from the floor and sat next to Mom on the bed.

"I have some bad news for you."

"What bad news?" I asked.

"Your Dad will not be with us anymore."

"How long will he be gone?" I asked.

Mom had tears in her eyes. "Forever, Jim."

During the next few days our family's activities were very busy. Shun and I were taken to Aunt Kate's house in the country. We were only gone a few days, but it seemed much longer.

Our trip home was warm and sunny. The sun's rays filled our living room with light that under other circumstances would have been cheerful. But as bright as it was, an emotional cloud darkened the room.

Passing my mourning relatives, I looked around and saw my dad asleep in his casket. I walked over and looked at him. My mother came and stood next to me. She placed her arm around my shoulder and said, "Your dad is gone, Jimmy."

With tears in my eyes and denial in my heart, I looked up at Mom and said, "You mean, forever?"

"Yes Jimmy, forever."

Finally, I accepted the unbelievable. I had not only lost my dad, I had lost my best friend. My heart was broken because the man I looked up to the most was gone. With a crushed spirit, I looked at Dad for the last time and walked away from the casket. I loved him so much and now he is with God.

This was the beginning of a long hard struggle for Mom. Dad had given her strength to carry on because she knew she would see him in Heaven one day. Mom lived with the faith that God would provide her with whatever she needed. This gave Mom the courage to take care of all of us.

My father's passing was a tremendous loss. The pain of having him one moment and gone the next was so intense that it felt as if someone had ripped my heart out of my body. Mom's major challenge was providing food and shelter for herself and six children, ranging in age from six months to fourteen years, one of whom had a severe physical disability. Mom had a rheumatic heart that made it more difficult to deal with this new situation, but she made whatever decisions were needed.

A friend of my father's once said to me, "If you're half the man your father was, you'll be someone special." I've always remembered this because it gave me a lofty goal. Even though

I'll never be the man Dad was, his example has given me the passion to strive for excellence. Someday when I go home to be with the Lord, He will say to me as He said to my dad, "Well done, Thou good and faithful servant."

Mom gave all six boys responsibilities: making the beds, dusting and sweeping, washing dishes, ironing clothes, doing the wash, hanging it out on the line, taking out the garbage, yard work, and whatever needed to be done. The older brothers made sure the younger ones did their jobs.

When Dad died, he owned two Clover Farm grocery stores, two ice cream parlors, and ran the Post Office in McGrann. After his death Mom sold the businesses to pay the bills and replaced Dad as the Postmaster.

We moved from our home to an apartment above the Post Office. It was a two bedroom apartment with a living room, dining room, and kitchen. It was just two blocks from our house, but in a less fashionable part of the town. People who lived on Front Street considered themselves in a better part of the town because of the sidewalks.

We moved because we were not able to afford our house any longer. After being in the house all of our lives, we didn't want to move, especially to a smaller place, but we had no other choice.

As difficult as this was for Mom, she never looked back. Her work at the Post Office provided a living for all of us. Mom's spirit wouldn't allow her to quit.

10

My friend John's garage was located about a half block from my home. It was big enough to park two large trucks, but the trucks were no longer there. It was a great place to play, especially when it was raining.

In the middle of the garage, a huge rope hung from the rafters and we took turns swinging on it. We pushed off a large chest full of clothes sitting in the middle of the room. This gave us a better swing around the garage. It was important that each person held onto the rope as tightly as possible. Hitting the chest with any part of the body caused a great deal of pain.

The rope was long and if the swingers were good enough, they used their feet to push off the wall to go faster. I was seven and a half and thought it was a lot of fun.

One time, I was in the garage by myself and played on the swing too long. My hands were tired and I had trouble holding onto the rope. I pushed off for my last swing before going home for supper. The rope circled the garage and when it came back to the center, my back faced the huge chest and my hands slipped.

My lower back hit the corner of the chest, near the soft spot located at my tailbone where my open hole had been, with the full impact of my weight. The force of my body hitting the chest caused severe damage to the spinal nerve which resulted in a major muscle spasm in my back. The blow knocked the wind out of me and when I tried to stand up to go home my legs didn't move. I was paralyzed from the waist down. The pain was excruciating and it took a long time before my legs were strong enough to support me to walk.

As soon as I came into the house bent over in pain, Mom could see something was wrong and called Dr. Winters. He could see the blow to my back was serious. Each time he touched the soft spot my legs gave out and I fell to the ground. That meant my back had to be protected so that nothing could hit it. My legs became weaker with each bump on the soft spot. The pressure of tapping a typewriter key was all it took to paralyze me.

After this I had to have someone with me when I swung on the rope. Since Tarzan was very popular in the movies, everyone took turns playing Tarzan, except me. My swing was more like a chimpanzee. We all had fun taking our turns. Of course, it wouldn't be a good swing without the Tarzan yell. We were pathetic, but we thought we sounded great.

"I'm Tarzan." The guys would swing and yell.

"I'm Jane," the girls yelled.

When it was my turn, I'd swing on the rope and make the sound of the chimp with his lips puckered up for a kiss and yell, "I'm Cheetah." It was good for laughs and with my long arms, and short body, if I had had more hair on my body, it would have been hard to tell us apart.

From this point on, every time that spot was bumped, it paralyzed me. After a while, my legs regained their strength and supported me as before. If that soft spot had been hit dead center, it would have paralyzed me from the waist down for the rest of my life. When I look back at what might have been I am reminded how fortunate I was. Things could have been much worse.

I have always tried to see my cup half full instead of half empty. Even though my legs became weaker and weaker with each bump on the soft spot, I tried to be thankful. Our minister said so many times, "You have to be thankful in everything." As a young kid, it was a lesson that was becoming more difficult for me to learn. I wanted to be able to do the same stunts as the other kids, but my body was not up to it, so I became increasingly cautious.

So many times my back felt like a hundred knives stuck all over it. With each movement, the penetration went deeper into my body. This caused my body to become very hot. It was like a high temperature, yet if anyone touched me, the person couldn't feel the heat. In the wintertime, I went outside in a T-shirt and wasn't cold. The pain was something that I had to work through, even though it was tough. It hurt whenever I'd walk or run, but this used up energy. Whether it was my imagination or not, my body seemed to cool off.

I'd say to the pain, "Nothing you do will take away my desire to walk. Whatever you throw at me, I'll come after you and you won't like that." My heart told me if I leaned on God, He may not give me relief, but He would be there for me when the pain became more intense. I never doubted my ability to shut off the pain. It was easy because I turned it over to God and He provided the strength for me to endure.

11

Due to my spina bifida, my legs were inverted to the center of my body, so my doctor had placed casts on my legs, trying to straighten out my feet. My brother Tug would carry me outside to sit when the weather was nice. The Post Office was located beneath our apartment and I'd greet everyone who came there.

In the late thirties, Big Foot worked the night shift at the factory. He rode with a friend who dropped him off in front of our home and he would visit me for a few minutes every day. During this time we became the best of friends.

At six feet tall and well over two hundred pounds, Big Foot was huge and strong as a bull. He was the kindest man I knew when he was sober. It was a different story when he was drunk. When drinking he was mean. No one did or said anything to make him angry because he'd start a fight. He had huge fists and if he ever hit anyone, the person would be picked up in another county for flying without a license.

Our relationship was special. He would encourage me by saying, "Jimmy, you're the toughest little guy I've ever known. Here you sit with casts up to your hips and you aren't mad. How can you be so happy when you have it so tough? You're really special, Jimmy."

He seemed pleased when I thanked him and said I love you too.

"Jimmy, don't get discouraged. If anyone can make it you're the one who will do it." Big Foot believed in me. He continued to encourage me whether anyone was around or not. Outside of my family, few people believed in me. Big Foot's encouragement gave me the desire to overcome my problems. His powerful love touched my heart.

One evening, after I was out of my casts, Big Foot sat in front of our house blocking traffic. Fearing he would hit Big Foot, the bus driver sat and waited.

I was playing with some friends and when we walked around to the front of my house, we saw Big Foot sitting in the middle of the road. People tried to move him, but he swung at anyone who came near him. When I saw Big Foot, I asked my mother if I could take Big Foot home.

Our minister, who was visiting with Mom, asked, "Aren't you afraid of him?"

"No. He'd never hurt me," I answered.

I walked over to where he was sitting and asked, "Big Foot, why are you sitting in the middle of the road?"

"I'm just resting," he answered.

"Why won't you allow the bus to go around you?"

"It can go around me, if it wants to." He didn't realize he was preventing the bus from moving past him.

A crowd had gathered in front of our home waiting to see what Big Foot was going to do. They were surprised when he didn't hit me.

"Let's go home, Big Foot."

"Okay Jimmy, I'm ready to go." He was having a difficult time standing up and staggered, almost falling.

"Big Foot, do you want me to help you get up?"

"No Jimmy, I'm too heavy for you."

Big Foot didn't think of me as a threat so he went along with me. I didn't walk very fast. That was okay because Big Foot didn't move very fast either. "Big Foot, give me your hand." He held it out and I grabbed a finger. His hands were so huge that my hand fit around his little finger perfectly.

People saw Big Foot as the town drunk and me as the town cripple. The crowd stayed a safe distance from us still expecting him to charge them if they came too close. Despite their fear they continued to follow us.

When we came around the corner across the street from Big Foot's house, we saw his wife, Kate standing on the porch. She looked relieved to see him coming home. With Big Foot's drinking she probably feared the police had taken him to jail. She thanked me for bringing him home and led him into the house.

That incident with Big Foot did in one evening what couldn't have been done in a lifetime. God showed the community what His true love was all about. The crowd saw how strong Big Foot's love was for me and how special he treated me. I knew without a doubt he'd never raise a hand to hurt me. He loved me too much for that.

Following this the community saw us in a different light. They saw the courage of a little boy, as well as the love of a big man. I didn't need courage when I was with someone who loved me. It must have impressed them because they treated both of us well after that. It was the first time people in the community saw my heart and not my disability. Whenever anyone looks inside a person's heart, God will show them a beautiful sight and it's a blessed gift.

12

My brother Tug was the quarterback and captain of the football team and his selection of plays always confused the opposing team. Shun and I enjoyed watching him play and we didn't miss any of his games.

Tug was tough and even played while injured. When I was nine, he suffered a dislocated shoulder in a game and wasn't able to move his right arm to throw a pass. Instead of dropping out, he stayed in the game and used his left hand to pass or hand the ball off. It took a great deal of concentration to play with such severe pain, but he was able to turn off the pain like flipping a light switch.

After the game we walked about half way up the sidewalk toward the gym and the players' entrance. This kid ran into us and knocked me to the ground. As he ran by he yelled, "Get outta my way, Crip." Shun was really angry and ran after him. He caught up with him and said, "I want you to apologize to my brother for knocking him down."

Lou was completely surprised when Shun challenged him. He didn't know who we were, but would soon learn Shun knew how to defend himself.

Lou made a sarcastic comment to Shun and said, "You don't want to mess with me. I'm a Golden Glove's boxing champion and you might get hurt."

They squared off. Lou was doing some fancy footwork and not paying attention to Shun. Thinking he knew all the moves to avoid being hit, he held the overconfident belief that no one could beat him. Up to this point no one had, especially in the ring. Lou was cocky and felt pretty big. His sarcastic comments made people angry, forcing them to defend themselves. Then Lou could show off his boxing skills and embarrass his victims.

He was used to doing whatever he wanted, with no one confronting him. If anyone challenged him, he would beat them up. He was a good fighter quick, smart, and sure-footed.

After a little while, he started watching Shun out of the corner of his eye. Shun realized what he was doing and faked a punch. Lou ducked and Shun punched hard right through his defense, knocking him off of his feet to the ground with a thud.

Other people waiting for the players formed a circle around them. Lou didn't get up right away. He just lay on the ground saying hateful things about me. Shun reached down, grabbed him by the front of his shirt, and lifted him to his feet. A repeated request for an apology was met with another smart remark, so Shun hit Lou again knocking him to the ground.

Lou picked himself up and started to do some fancy footwork. He'd jab, then feint and duck, dancing into Shun's reach and out again looking at his friends. During this performance his face wore a smirk of contempt.

Once when Lou swung and missed, Shun hit him with a shot to the chin that knocked him down again. It happened so fast Lou didn't know what hit him or where the punch came from. Shun had had enough of his smart mouth, so he picked him up again and demanded, "You are going to apologize to my brother Jim."

Lou was humiliated because he lost to someone who had had no boxing experience. Shun was not a fighter, but when provoked he would stand up for what he felt was right. When Lou hit me from behind, Shun was disgusted and would not tolerate this outrage.

Finally Lou apologized to me and was really embarrassed. Many years later, after Lou and I became good friends, he told me he was glad he apologized.

13

When one of my "friends" was angry about something and took his anger out on me, it wasn't very nice. While he was yelling at me I said, "Your sweater looks nice on you."

This surprised the kid and frustrated him because he wanted to knock my block off. My goal was to keep the block on my shoulders.

"What did you say?" he asked. After repeating my statement, he said something under his breath and walked away. This really surprised me, because he was heading for a fight. His reaction pleased me so much, I ran home and told my mother what I had done. When he saw me later, his reaction was much kinder. I thought, "Maybe, if I'm honest, this kindness will work." When I say something nice, I'm not looking to hurt anyone and a kind word makes the other person feel good from within. This was one of the ways for me to rise above it. Gradually, this little kid was going to grow up.

The prejudice expressed by the kids diminished. This incident and my use of humor were two of the reasons many people in the community looked on me with less scorn. There were some who could not look past my physical disability, to see there was a human being inside this disabled body, but they didn't have a chance, because of my successful use of humor. Telling someone they looked nice, enabled me to win them over with love. I cannot take credit for this, the thought came from

God. I would have to stand up to more ridicule, but now the tide was turning and God placed confidence in my heart and mind. Someday, whenever those who can't see past the disability finally see what God has done, they won't forget that my difference came from God.

Whenever people are mean and the victim responds with kindness, it opens the person's eyes and they will feel bad about what they said.

14

Pain was a great teacher. It helped me to develop a good foundation for improving my attitude. It didn't happen at once and sometimes there was no progress at all. Other times, there was a little improvement or even major strides. This only happened after a long fight with the problem and I learned how to develop a more thoughtful attitude while improving the situation. Major changes occurred when I couldn't overcome a problem and had to learn to live with it. Learning this was a major accomplishment that in the long run made me a better person. Whether I was swimming, biking, or hiking, I learned not to quit. I replaced complaining with humor directed at myself and never used it to hurt anyone else. I wanted people to see that I didn't take myself too seriously.

Whenever the pain became intense, it was evident by the deep lines in my face, next to my nose, and down toward my lips. Sometimes a caring adult would hurt for me as well and turn away in tears, having seen God's spirit in my heart. The thoughtful consideration by these beautiful people increased my desire to fight my pain without complaining and not allow it to consume me. My fight to cope with the pain was a continual one. So many times the pain was way ahead. The intensity of it made me work a little harder to catch up, which took quite a while. It never occurred to me that the community respected me because they saw God's love.

The muscle spasms started at the base of my neck. The pressure felt like someone squeezed the back of my neck with a pipe wrench. My head was so sensitive to touch that rubbing it increased the pain. My shoulders were drawn toward the center of my body and my chest was pulled down toward the diaphragm. Spasms continued down my spine causing my ribs to tighten and prevented natural breathing. My breath came in short gasps, like I was hyperventilating. The pressure on my lower back was so severe it felt like lava going through my veins and my hips felt like bone rubbing bone. The excruciating pain traveled down my legs which started to buckle as I dragged them along trying to walk. When I tried to stand up straight, I felt my body was at war with itself, with severe stiffness from head to toe. I treated this tightness the same as ridicule. I challenged the pain as if it were a person by saying, "You're not going to beat me." Standing up against it gave me a stronger desire to work toward some relief.

While bathing I learned that soaking in hot water released a lot of pressure from the muscles spasms. I filled the tub until the water reached the back of my neck, an area of major pain. I was able to move my neck from side to side and felt a lot less discomfort. Once my neck relaxed, I'd soak a towel in hot water then place it on top of my head. The heat relieved the vice-like pressure and softened the pounding in my temples. Next, I'd place the hot towel on my face. The heat eased my double vision and I was able to focus. The little man inside my head pushing my eyeballs out was gone. I wasn't dizzy or light-headed anymore. My eyes didn't tear and became less bleary. The heat relaxed my chest and shoulders allowing me to breathe more easily. Without the severe burning sensation in my lower back and hips and with the excruciating pain gone from my legs, I was able to stand and walk. I would soak in the tub for a half hour in the evening. It was the only way to relax my body enough to cope with the severe pain.

I was able to sleep through most of the night and get through part of the day before the severe pressure returned. In the beginning, I fought the pain when I was exhausted and was never able to stay even with it. Knowing when to rest gave me more energy for the fight.

I would rub and stretch my muscles until the spasms relaxed and I was able to move. Movement became easier with decreased pain, but the effort took its toll on my attitude. I carried this burden like a five hundred-pound weight on my shoulders. The weight was too heavy for me until God provided relief, giving me a more positive outlook.

First it was up to me to show the community I was worthy of respect. I would use a softer approach with others while standing up for myself. Second, I'd work on my bad attitude by treating others the way I wanted to be treated. This was the only way the community would see a difference in me.

My negative attitude was difficult to live with because it showed me how defeated a person can feel. The worthless feeling in my heart didn't allow God to show His love for me. It is easy to dwell on what's wrong rather than working to find a way to make the bad attitude a positive one.

If I failed to make any adjustment to the pain and did not try to look for other solutions then I'd accept failure. I've always felt that if I didn't try I didn't deserve to succeed.

My reason for leaning on God so much wasn't so others would see how godly I was, it was a matter of survival. The positive attitude provided an opening for God to come into my heart and change this terrible negative feeling. A positive attitude must come from God. To solve our problems, we must be willing to share them with God. It means turning it all over to Him and allowing Him to help us work through the problem. These thoughts must be kept in mind when dealing with pain. If we lean on God, He'll provide the care, understanding and especially the love.

15

Dr. Winters had been searching for new ideas to develop strength in my muscles and to help straighten out my feet. He wanted me to have as normal a life as possible and my inverted feet might cause problems if they were not straightened. I was nine years old in 1940 when Dr. Winters learned about a new procedure in a medical journal. Cleveland Clinic had been developing the new procedure and was looking for candidates for the treatment. Dr. Winters wanted to see if I would be a good candidate, so he wrote and asked if I could have an interview.

I was young enough that this was probably the best time for me to have the surgery. Dr. Winters told them all about me in great detail. He thought my muscles were strong enough to make the surgery successful. My legs had to be reasonably strong for the muscles to hold my feet in place. Frequent running and walking gave me enough strength to qualify for the surgery.

When he received an invitation, Dr. Winters and Mom decided we should make the trip to Cleveland for the examination. Dr. Winters said we had nothing to lose and was pleased with the invitation. He felt the possibility of straightening my feet was an opportunity we couldn't pass up. He thought we should do anything to improve my inverted feet.

At first, I wasn't in favor of going back to the hospital. When this new opportunity was explained to me and the possible outcome, I changed my mind and was willing to accept it. With my feet straight in front of me, I would no longer be tripping over myself and I'd be able to move more normally. The doctors wanted this experimental procedure to become standard and we prayed that God would allow the operation to be successful. I was one of a number of candidates and blessed that my muscle tone was strong enough to insure success. Even more important than my being the first to have this operation was that many young people would have the same opportunity. It meant that God would be able to touch a lot of young people through this new procedure.

The doctors at Cleveland Clinic had shown a lot of interest in me by returning a positive letter to Dr. Winters. They felt there wasn't a better candidate for the new procedure and if successful, it would make a difference in my life.

The letter indicated the examination would take four to six hours. I was one of the candidates and no one had been selected yet. The right candidate had to be chosen because if the procedure failed, this new idea would have to be abandoned. It never entered my mind that I wouldn't be selected.

We had to travel to Cleveland from our home, about fifty miles north of Pittsburgh. Even though the trip was one hundred fifty miles each way, we didn't mind because the surgery could change my life. Mom hadn't gone ten miles when I asked, "Are we there, yet?" To a little boy of ten, this was a long trip.

When we finally reached our destination, I was awed by the busy four-lane highways. I came from a town of 1,500 people and Cleveland was the biggest city I'd ever seen.

We went to Cleveland Clinic with high hopes that this new procedure would be the answer to our prayers. At least we had received an invitation for me to be examined by the doctors. It was now up to them to determine if my muscles were strong enough for the operation.

We finally arrived for the appointment and Mom had to fill out a lot of papers detailing what had been done. She felt that whatever happened, Dr. Winters had found the place where we should be. When she finished the paperwork the doctors requested, we were asked to come back the next day for the examination.

We arrived at the hospital early only to wait, and wait, and wait. A nurse took us into the examining room later that morning. The room was very small, but large enough for me to do what they asked. Six doctors came to examine me and determine whether I would be a good candidate for the surgery. Their expressions were intense and they meant business.

The doctors took their time to assess my condition. If they had questions, the problems had to be worked out. Apparently, there weren't any problems because the decision was made quickly.

They took turns seeing what I could do. I was pushed, pinched, and pulled. They asked me to stand, sit, bend, twist, stretch, walk and turn around. I did everything they asked. The doctors checked out every angle of my body. They had to be sure my muscles were strong enough to hold my feet in place. After the examination, they decided I would have the surgery. From that point on, everything moved very quickly. It was such a relief to get away from those doctors and have the exam behind me.

Following this demanding examination, arrangements were made to place me in the children's ward. I was tired and looking forward to this. The doctors had treated me very well, but I just wanted to lie down, even if it was in a hospital bed.

It felt great to have been chosen for the operation. That might sound strange, but the end result could change my life. Still I was frightened to be so far from home. The hospital was a quiet place when I arrived and I decided I was going to have some fun. This hospital wasn't going to prevent me from enjoying myself. My mother always said, "No matter how bad it is, have fun. It will take your mind off the problem. You'll have a better outlook. Stay positive and you won't be dwelling on how serious the situation is. It's important to be happy and enjoy yourself." I've always tried to put this into practice. It didn't occur to me that a positive attitude would help the surgery be successful.

The doctors wanted to see how my feet needed to be straightened. They needed x-rays to determine how to correct them. So a couple of days after my examination I was taken to X-ray in a wheelchair.

There was a little girl, about my age sitting next to me in a wheelchair. I tried to talk to her, even sing, but she ignored me and didn't smile. She was concentrating on her problem and didn't hear me. I'd tell her a joke, but the only laughter came from me.

I started looking down at the floor but she still ignored me. So I leaned a little farther out of my wheelchair. Finally, she looked at me and asked, "What are you doing?"

"I lost something," I answered. "Will you help me find it?" We both looked at the floor. I would look up at her and then back to the floor. The lost look and deep frown left her face, replaced by a desire to find whatever I had lost.

Slowly a grin came over her face and she said, "You know, we're looking for something, but you didn't tell me what we're looking for." She still had a grin on her face. "Did you lose something or didn't you?" I didn't say anything to her. The grin on my face made her laugh. Her nose wrinkled and a big smile came across her face.

I looked down at the floor and back at her and said, "Hey, I found it. It was right here in front of me. I just didn't see it."

She looked at me and asked, "If it was in front of you, why didn't you see it?"

I looked at her bright eyes and pretty smile and answered, "I was looking for your smile and thought it was on the floor. That's where your chin was so your smile had to be there too."

She made a comment that really fit me when she said, "You know, you're a nut."

"Well, you know, when I was singing to you, I was totally ignored. So, I asked you to dance and you still ignored me."

"We're both in wheelchairs, how can we dance?"

"We can dream can't we?"

She shared her fears about what was going to happen to her. Her burden was heavy. "Life is here to enjoy," I told her. "We have to make the most of it. Don't allow sickness to get in the way of being happy and having fun. If you're happy you can make your life better and turn away the bad thoughts. Hang in there, enjoy the moment for what it's worth, and don't waste it." She smiled at me and left. That was good advice coming from a smart aleck kid.

She had to be reached, but it was difficult because of her painful thoughts. She was hurting inside and needed someone to lighten her load and relax her heart. It had to be a nut, loose in a wheelchair, and I fit the description to a T.

Pain can be so devastating that it requires all your energy to deal with it. Once it starts to consume a person, it's very difficult to regain a positive attitude. Humor can allow people to forget about how bad they feel for a few minutes. This can be a great service. I thought it was so sad how the pain and fear had stolen that pretty little girl's smile. It had to be replaced somehow by a nutty kid.

God used this special feeling to make me feel warm inside. That little girl's pleasant response was so remarkable that it fueled my desire to reach out and touch someone else's heart to make their day just a little brighter for a few minutes. If I can make someone feel good by acting like a nut, it's worth the effort.

That was the last time I saw her. I don't know if my actions made any difference, but the smile on her face gave her a few minutes away from her severe problems. This began what I've always tried to do, make someone laugh and enjoy the moment.

16

It was lonely in the hospital where Mom was my only visitor. At home there was always someone to play with, but here in the hospital, there were only the other children in the ward.

Loneliness always came when I felt sorry for myself. I wanted the kids in the ward to have a good time and it was up to me to start it. Anyone who walked into our ward had an instant friend, me. It didn't matter who they were, I'd talk to them. I had never met a stranger in my life and it wasn't going to start now. I believe this spirit came from God. He placed that feeling in my heart. I knew that His love made me someone special and I have always believed this.

My family had never said anything about my life being close to the edge, that it was possible for me to go home to be with the Lord any day. Even though no one said it, I had the feeling my life had to be lived each day as if it were my last. My pain was so severe that whenever I had some relief, I'd enjoy the day to the fullest. It was up to me to make the most out of each day. My physical disability didn't need to be pointed out; my pain reminded me of it every day.

Shortly after the x-rays were read, I was taken to surgery. "You'll go to sleep shortly," the doctor said.

"Doc, I'm four foot eight, I go everywhere shortly." He just smiled and that's the last thing I remember.

During the surgery, I dreamed of being back at home under the bridge, standing in the middle of the creek. It was spring and we had a lot of rain. A flood was coming from the nearby hills. My foot was stuck under a huge rock. I tried to pull it free. The water continued coming down from the hills into this small creek. People were watching and gave me the exact location of the floodwaters.

My body was jumping and twisting until I landed on the operating table. I'm sure it was difficult for my dream surgeons to operate on a yoyo moving up and down.

The more I pulled on my foot, the tighter the doctors clamped it down. My foot under the clamp was the same one under the huge rock in the creek. The tightness of the clamp caused me to twist and turn my body on the operating table.

The floodwaters were on top of me and I still wasn't able to move. I yelled at the top of my voice, "Get me outta here!" The doctors in my dream jumped about a foot in the air and finished the surgery when their feet hit the ground.

While in recovery, the doctors told me how difficult the operation was, though it was easy compared to my dream. They asked me, "Jimmy, what were you dreaming about?" I shared my experience with them. "Well Jimmy, we all had quite an experience, didn't we?"

This surgery was a success. The doctors worked hard and God had His hand on the surgeons. They were pleased with the results. Everything they tried was successful and my muscles were strong enough to hold my feet straight in front of me.

Following my recovery, an orderly wheeled me back to the children's ward. I felt a little groggy and had no feeling from the waist down. I wondered where my legs and feet were.

I yelled to a nurse standing by my bed, "Okay, What did you do with them? I had them when I came in here."

"Did with what?" she asked.

"Where did you put my legs?"

The nurse grinned and answered, "Your legs are under the metal tent which prevents you from moving them."

"You mean my legs and feet are camping out and I have to stay in the hospital?"

The nurse laughed. "Yes, that's what it looks like. You'll get used to it." She smiled and walked away.

Genny was the prettiest nurse I'd ever seen. She had auburn hair, soft white skin, and a beautiful smile. Her eyes were always smiling and her friendly disposition helped us all relax in the ward. Genny loved young people. Each of us believed Genny was our girlfriend and we all loved her. It didn't matter that we didn't know what love was. Talk about puppy love, our hearts barked for attention when she came into the ward.

She treated each one of us as if we were the most important person in her life. We couldn't wait until she came into our ward. Everyone greeted her at once and shared something with her. She always listened until the person finished talking to her. Genny's attention helped us to think about her and not why we were in the hospital. We were not lonely because of her interest in us.

If anyone asked Genny for something we weren't allowed to have, she took the time to explain why the doctors didn't permit it.

It was especially tough on me because I had to lie still. I'm not one to be in the same place twice. The tent was a great way for the doctors to keep an eye on me and it worked. The tent had me confined, but it didn't quiet my tongue. My jaws continued moving up and down constantly and it still hasn't changed. The pain in my lower back was severe because of the pressure on my soft spot, but I wasn't able to move. This was the first step to straighten my feet and I kept a positive outlook, thinking of all the fun I'd have.

Mom was staying in a motel near the hospital and came to visit me every day. She would bring me something to play with or to read. This helped me keep busy while staying in the hospital. The books suited me and I could read them quickly. When reading the stories, I'd concentrate so hard on the main character that I'd take his place in my mind. It helped me to live someone else's life while being cooped up in a hospital. Reading helped me step outside my body and be someone free of pain.

This was the beginning of a new life for me. Up to this time, I did not do much reading. It was a nice feeling to read and forget about the pain that was with me constantly. After I finished reading or working or playing with whatever Mom brought me, I'd pass it around the ward to the other young people. If we shared what was given to us, I learned we could improve our relationships.

Well past midnight, a couple of nights after the tent was removed, I tossed and turned most of the night. In the background a car horn was stuck and the loud noise bothered me. The night nurse was sitting in a chair leaning against the wall reading the paper. The two back legs of his chair touched the floor with the front legs in the air. I yelled so loud it made him jump and when he came down and landed on the chair, he lost his balance and fell to the floor.

He came over to my bed to see if I was okay. He told me what had happened and we both laughed. I don't think he leaned his chair against the wall in our ward again. It's funny how you can cure people of doing that.

I looked forward to these trips out of the children's ward regardless of what was going to be done. The time away from the ward helped me to pass the time and gave me the opportunity to see other places in the hospital. I was also eager to have my casts removed. Dr. Winters had done this so many times in the past that I expected my feet to still be inverted. To my surprise my feet remained pointed straight ahead.

My feet were dirty, smelly, and the dry skin made my feet itch. They were caked with dried blood so black my feet looked decayed. To the average observer I'm sure my scarred feet looked terrible. Yet to me, it was the most beautiful sight I'd ever seen. I wasn't able to take my eyes off my feet.

The doctor washed my feet as gently as he could. The skin was tender and it didn't take much pressure to cause my feet to bleed. The washing softened the stitches and the coolness of the water felt great.

After cleaning my feet, the doctor soaked the stitches to make them easier to cut. He lifted each stitch with tweezers, cut it in the middle and removed it. There were one hundred fifty stitches in each foot and they all had to be removed.

Since the hair on my legs was the same color as the stitches, sometimes the doctor would pull what he thought was a stitch, but got a hair instead. When this happened I'd say, "Do you mind Doc? Cut the stitches not the hair." The doctor laughed. He'd remove a couple of stitches and start laughing again.

When the doctor removed my stitches at the hospital, he put new casts on my feet. I would have to wear them at home for six months, because I was not allowed to stand or put any weight on my feet.

The removal of the stitches meant I'd be going home in a few days. My stay in the hospital was a good one. Even confined to bed, my life was fun and no one seemed to tire of me. The surgery was successful which meant walking would be much easier. Closing my eyes I could see myself running a race with other kids and keeping up with them. It was the most beautiful vision and a blessing from God.

I looked at my feet and remembered how bad they looked before the surgery. Now with both feet in front of me, it was the greatest feeling I'd ever experienced. It was hard to believe my feet were going to be normal. I thought about all the times the kids chased me because of my disability. I wasn't able to run fast enough to escape my tormentors. With straight feet I'd be able to defend myself and play games with the other kids. I just wanted to be a little more normal, though I've never been accused of that.

This was an opportunity to start my life anew. I would be able to push myself up out of a chair and stand on my feet without falling. I just wanted to run as well as any other kid, to play in games and not be the last one picked for the teams.

With my inverted feet I lacked balance and the ability to control my legs. I didn't have the strength to pick up my feet when I walked. As a result, I'd trip and fall when the front of my foot couldn't clear a crack in the cement, or a stone caused me to slip.

My balance would improve with my feet straight out in front of me. However, it would be many months before I'd have the opportunity to try out my new feet. The healing took a lot of time, but the doctor's approval for me to start walking was worth waiting for.

Toward the end of the second week, after the stitches had been removed the doctor came to see me with the biggest grin on his face. "Would you like to go home?" He was always kind and considerate, taking great pleasure in doing something nice for me. If I didn't understand something, he would explain it in a different way and never talked over my head.

"How would you like to go home?" he asked me again. I looked around thinking he was talking to someone else.

"Are you talking to me?" I wasn't expecting him to ask me about going home.

"Yes Jimmy, I'm talking to you."

"Well doctor, I don't want to rush you. Is it okay to go now? Do you really mean it?"

"Yes, I mean it."

"Does my mother know? If she doesn't, may I tell her?"

"I haven't seen your mother yet. Yes you may tell her."

Since I was leaving, the doctor stayed longer to talk to me. "What do you think of our hospital?" he asked.

"Don't eat the food, it might make you sick and then you'd have to go to the hospital," I whispered. "A hospital is not my favorite place to stay. You can give it back to the Indians-- Cleveland Indians, that is."

He laughed and stood up ready to leave. "I'm going to miss you, Jimmy. You're a tough little guy. Don't lose your desire to fight back." He reached out and shook my hand.

Mom came in later and I told her what the doctor had said. His words of encouragement were special. I would miss him but I was very eager to go home. I had been away only a couple of weeks, but I still wondered if anyone back home missed me.

Everyone here seemed to know who I was. If they didn't, I'd tell them, "I'm Jim Byron." Everyone was happy for me because I was going home. All my friends at the hospital came in and wished me well. I was surprised that everyone seemed to like me. Back home I had very few friends, but here we treated each other with kindness and respect. It was important for me to show my new friends that I really cared. This was easy for me, having been brought up in a family that had always done this so well. I'm an expert because I'm the one who received the most care and always with love. I wanted to pass on what was given to me and do it without expecting anything in return.

The next day Mom came early to help me dress for the trip home. As soon as she walked into the room, I was ready. It seemed like it took forever for them to check me out of the hospital. As I left many people came out to see me off. In that short time I'd made so many nice friends. I'd say to anyone who listened, "Hi, I'm Jim Byron. I'm going home today." No, I wasn't excited about it. I was ecstatic. When ignored, I'd yell and tell them I was going home. Talk about an ego trip, I was on a big one.

After we left the hospital, I sat in the back seat of our car with my legs extended across the seat. We had not gone very far when a car crossed in front of us without any warning. When Fred, a family friend who offered to drive us home, stepped on the brakes, the momentum threw me to the floor. Fearing I might have been hurt or my casts broken, he stopped the car to check, but I was more scared than hurt. The trip home was a long one and I was exhausted. So I wasn't very talkative. I just wanted to go home. When we pulled into our driveway, it was the most satisfying feeling I'd ever known.

Sometimes my friend Junior would visit. He was nice to me for a little while and then would start to read my new comic books. When he finished reading them he would leave. If he came again and I didn't have any new comic books, he would say a couple of words and go home. It was good to have the company even if reading my comic books was all he wanted to do. When my brother Tug saw Junior paying so little attention to me he asked, "Did you come to see Jim?"

"Yes," he answered.

"Put the comic books down, now." After a while Tug came back into the room and saw Junior still reading a comic book. He took it out of his hand and escorted him to the door. "Don't come back unless you are going to visit with Jim. You will not come here just to read his comic books. You'll either visit with him, or you won't come back." I was pleased with Tug's willingness to stand up for me. Even though that was Junior's last visit, I thought Tug was the greatest.

Tug carried me everywhere--downstairs, then upstairs to this room and that room. He helped me down on the floor to play with my toy soldiers. My casts were heavy and I was surprised at how easily he was able to pick up such a heavy load.

One day, when Tug was carrying me downstairs, he lost his balance and we fell down about eight or ten steps to the bottom of the stairs. Since Tug was in front of me, my casts hit him on the head at each step. His head must have been ringing. Finally, when we landed at the bottom of the stairs, Tug jumped up and asked if I was all right. "How's your head?" I asked him. "Does it hurt from all the banging from my casts?"

"I'm all right," Tug said.

I thought to myself, "Boy, he has a hard head." I used to tease him by saying the reason he had so many problems was because my cast hit him on the head so hard. He always had the ability to rise above any tough situations.

As I look back on the special care Tug gave me, I'm reminded how fortunate I was to have brothers who loved me so much. It was not stated as much as continually shown.

Six months later, when I returned to Cleveland Clinic for a follow-up exam, the doctor examined my feet and replaced the old casts with new ones. He attached steel pegs about two and a half inches long to the casts at the middle of each foot. A rubber cap slipped over the metal peg to give me the traction I needed and prevented my feet from slipping out from under me when I walked.

So six months after my surgery, at age ten and a half, the doctor said it was okay for me to start walking. I'd been sitting for the last year without any pressure on my feet. Learning to walk again was a very slow process. No one told me how. I was just expected to do it. This was the beginning of a difficult though wonderful experience.

When the weather was nice, Tug would take me and my chair outside our apartment to an area next to the barber shop to practice. The ability to stand up without holding the arms of the chair was won inch by inch. At first I noticed no change in my attempts to push myself out of the chair. It took a number of attempts just to lift myself. I'd push up until my arms were fully extended. Many times my arms tired and I'd fall back into the chair. This fueled my desire to do it again.

After practicing I would give a stronger push then sit and rest before another attempt. Whenever I was able to push myself a little higher, the milestone was etched in my mind. I worked to build my strength and continued until my legs held me up and I was able to stand. The effort exhausted me, yet the fear of spending the rest of my life in a wheelchair gave me the incentive to continue trying.

I fought the tough battle because walking like everyone else was my first priority. I would accept nothing less. My strong faith helped me reach my goal. I just needed to develop my muscles to hold myself in an upright position and eventually my arms became stronger.

It took a long time to reach a standing position. Sometimes my legs could not hold me and I'd fall back into the chair. I would land with a hard painful thud which shook me from head to toe. Following a long period of inactivity, my energy had not been stretched to this point of exhaustion for some time. My arms and shoulders ached.

Extending my foot with my toes pointed straight in front of me was painful. Stretching the new skin made the top of my foot super sensitive. The burning sensation was so intense it felt like someone lit a match and threw it on my foot. This drained my energy, sapping my desire to walk.

After a little while I became brave again. Releasing my hold on the chair, I tried to stand without any support and I fell to the ground. I picked myself up and rested before starting again, with the same results. Every muscle in my body ached.

God used the pain to increase my determination. It made me angry and helped me focus on my goal of walking.

There was no way my life was going to be spent in a wheelchair. I'd walk with crutches if necessary. I wanted to have the freedom to go wherever I wanted. This meant I wouldn't have to wait for someone to carry me or push a wheelchair. My stubbornness was too strong for that to happen.

It took a long time to develop the strength to stand and maintain my balance. Finally when my legs became strong enough to support me, I took my first step.

There were cinders all around the side of our house because it was used as a parking lot for the barbershop next door. Each time I fell, my body landed on the cinders. My clothes were dirty as well as my arms and legs.

It wasn't until I started to examine what caused me to fall that I made some progress. I'd check to see if my balance was steady before releasing my grip from the chair. I didn't push away from the chair too hard, which would cause me to lose my balance. I'd check the ground to see where the cinders were. If I rocked forward on the steel pegs in the middle of each foot, my toes would hit the cinders and this hurt for a long time.

At first, I fell, got up, fell again, took another step, and fell once more. I repeated this over and over. After a long time my hands and legs were raw from falling on the ground so much. All I could think of was that darn wheelchair and I kept trying.

Before my next step, I saw some stones in my path. Not wanting to step on the stones, I shortened my step to miss them. At once, I noticed the pain was not nearly as intense. Later I lost my balance and did a couple stutter steps, stepping from side to side to maintain my balance. The short choppy stutter steps were a lot less painful. I was able to run like this better than I could walk.

This was a great accomplishment. Satisfaction warmed my heart and made my whole body glow. I now knew without a doubt I was free from the wheelchair. I had finally made it. Now I could enjoy the privilege of walking and the freedom that comes with this gift from God. Wow! What a blessing.

17

By the time I was thirteen my feet had healed nicely. The doctor at Cleveland Clinic who performed my operation thought it was time to replace my casts with orthopedic shoes. With heavy steel shanks to hold my feet in place, the new shoes would help strengthen my ankles. After wearing knee-high casts for three years, I was pleased to switch to shoes and I was excited when Mom took me to Pittsburgh to talk to a man about making them.

When my shoes were ready a couple of weeks later, Mom and I took the train back to Pittsburgh about fifty miles away to pick them up. While we were walking down the street in Pittsburgh, I was running alongside my mother just to keep up with her. Mom never wasted a moment and when she walked it was difficult for me to stay next to her. Mom had three speeds: drive, overdrive, and supersonic drive. To me, she always was in supersonic drive. She was the fastest lady on two feet I'd ever seen. In fact, she walked so fast that I don't think her feet touched the ground. After a while, I ran out of energy. Mom continued walking down the street talking to the person she thought was by her side, but it wasn't me. She sure looked funny talking to herself. I was sitting on a fire hydrant about a block and a half behind her when Mom finally realized I wasn't next to her. She looked back down the block, saw me, and came back to ask, "What are you doing?"

"I'm resting. Mom, you walk so fast I just can't keep up, even when I'm running by your side." Mom just laughed and slowed down for about a block.

My new shoes had strong steel braces attached to the heels that went up each side of the shoe to my knees. There were straps attached to the top of the braces that went around my leg, just below the knee. This also took some of the weight off my feet to prevent me from falling. I'm sure it really looked terrible to wear braces, but it was great to be out of the casts and these were the most beautiful shoes I'd ever seen. They were mine.

The man who made my shoes was named Fritz. He was a very gentle person who had a great sense of humor. His kindness went a long way in developing a great friendship. He went the extra steps to make sure the shoes were comfortable. Fritz never gave up on finding what had to be done to help me enjoy my new shoes.

I could have griped about the pain, but no one wants to be around anyone who talks about how bad they feel. I don't want to be around anyone like that either. This was another adjustment that had to be made without complaining.

Fritz told me it might take a while to find the right adjustment so the shoes wouldn't hurt. "These shoes will make a dramatic change in your feet, but could cause a great deal of pain."

The new shoes were stiff with very little give, which prevented my toes from bending when I walked. The seams rubbed my feet raw and caused my toes to become very tender. My feet throbbed for a couple of weeks and kept me awake at night. The pain was so intense I wanted to cut my feet off at the ankles.

Fritz padded the area where the seams were, to make it easier for me to walk. I knew Fritz was doing everything he could to help me adjust. Each time the shoes fit just a little better than the last time. Fritz made a special piece of leather that fit at the bottom of both shoes behind my toes. He felt this was the best place for the leather because it automatically caused my feet to bend forward and forced me to walk on my toes. Eventually the stretching became much easier. This took a lot of the soreness out of my toes and made it easier for me to stretch them and make them stronger.

The modifications didn't take away from the natural beauty of the shoes. I was proud when I started wearing my new shoes. They were nice looking, unlike the original clodhoppers that caused me to bump my toes so often, hurt my feet, and shot pain all the way to my hips. It was a nice feeling to have shoes on my feet which were not painful to put on, even if there were braces attached.

After finally arriving home, I went all over our community telling anyone who would listen about my new shoes. Even if they didn't know me, they knew about the shoes. If people thought I was crazy, my incessant talking about my shoes proved them right.

18

In McGrann, our grade school was referred to as McGrann University or Bellwood Pre-Flight. Most of the kids who went to Bellwood were real characters. When we talked to other kids about our school, they thought we were going to college. Then we would explain to them that this is what our grade school was called.

The building was very old. When the weather was cold and we had freezing rain, sometimes the pipes would break. When this happened, school would be called off for the day and the kids were happy.

The outer walls of the building had white cement about five feet high on all sides. I was fourteen when some of the boys in the upper grades found some colored chalk and wrote some graffiti all over the lower walls of the building.

The next morning the principal came into our room and asked if any of us knew who had been writing all over the building. One of the kids in our class said he saw me outside the building yesterday.

"Jimmy, were you on the school grounds yesterday?" the principal asked.

"Yes, I was there last night."

"Jimmy, did you write on the school wall?"

"No, I didn't."

"Do you know who did?"

"No. I saw the writing, but no one was around."

A couple of days later, after the principal checked on our stories, the boys who remained under suspicion were told to stand. "You're going to be spanked in front of your classmates." The principal marched all of them to the front of the room. "This is what happens when you damage the school."

Our principal was a very big woman, who stood close to six feet tall and weighed two hundred pounds with very little fat on her. She had worked on a farm all her life and was so tough that you didn't want to make her angry. Though she was hard on you when you did something wrong, she was fair in her judgment.

Starting with the first person she asked, "Did you write on the building?" She had a two-inch paddle, with half-inch holes to make it sting a little more on contact. I'll tell you this, I'm happy that I wasn't one of the kids receiving the spanking. Our principal looked like she was at the plate batting, swinging for the fences trying for a home run. She convinced all of us that we didn't want a spanking from her. Those who received a spanking weren't able to sit down for a while.

She worked down the line, spanking each of her victims. They showed no emotion, but you could see in their eyes they felt each swing.

Jim was last in line. Each time the principal hit him with the paddle, he jumped about two or three inches off the ground. We all laughed, because we thought Jim was trying to be funny. He screamed with each hit. You could hear him all over the school. After the spanking was over the principal said, "You may go back to your seat and sit down."

"I'll go back to my seat," he said, "but I'm not sitting down."

Thinking he was being disrespectful she said, "You're going to do what you're told."

"Well, I'd like to, but I had a two-inch bolt in my pocket when you spanked me. My bottom hurts and I can't sit on it. Every time you hit me, you drove the bolt deeper into my bottom. I tried to get it out, but you swung the paddle so fast you hit my fingers." She laughed along with the whole room. It relieved the tension we all felt.

From then on every time she saw him, she just smiled. Jim was teased for a long time about the bolt in his pocket. This was a good lesson for everyone, because no one ever wrote on the school walls again. Jim would never forget the incident and neither would I

You never wanted our principal against you. She demanded respect and wasn't one to hold a grudge. Whenever she spoke to you, you had better answer her with respect. She knew that if she asked me a question, I would give her an honest answer. I admired her and we became good friends.

19

When I was fourteen, Shun took me over to the baseball field near McGrann to teach me how to field grounders. At first most of the grounders bounced off my glove and rolled toward the outfield. I'd try to field each grounder, following the ball with my glove and close my eyes at the last moment, just as the ball came toward me. Most balls that hit my glove did not remain there. Instead they bounced off the glove and hit me in the nose. Each time Shun reminded me to keep my eye on the ball. Finally, after all my mistakes, it was time to try Shun's suggestion. I'd watch the ball, follow it, and catch it in my glove.

Whenever the ball slipped through my glove, I'd say to Shun, "I must have a hole in my glove, otherwise, how did it get through?"

Shun laughed. "Well, you need to plug that hole."

Gradually, my fielding improved with a lot of practice. I was able to field the ball and throw it back to Shun in one motion. My concentration on the ball became so strong that I'd follow it, whether it stayed down low, hit a stone, bounced high, or came at my feet in a line drive. If I couldn't make a play with the ball, I'd try to knock it down and keep it in front of me. This would prevent a runner from getting an extra base. Shun's willingness to correct my mistakes taught me to be an excellent fielder. Whenever I made a mistake, Shun took the time to show me what caused it. "If you had moved this way you would have made the play." His instructions were responsible for much of my success. My failures occurred when I was out of position to field the ball.

Shun also taught me how to catch pop flies or any ball hit into the air. When he hit the ball straight up, it seemed to stay in the air forever. I'd stagger under the ball, trying to gauge where it would come down. If anyone had seen me, they would have thought I was trained by a chimpanzee that stepped on a banana peel.

"I get dizzy, looking up in the sky trying to catch fly balls," I told Shun.

"You were dizzy long before looking up into the sky."

Shun was an excellent athlete, with tremendous strength and agility, who intimidated his opponents. One never knew what he was going to do. He was so quick that when he faked one way, by the time you responded he was gone.

Shun always showed me how to improve what I was doing. He taught me to look for solutions. He said, "Watch how the batter positions his feet. That will tell you what field he is hitting to. Move to where you think the ball will be hit. This way you will move less and be able to make the play."

When I first played the game, I wasn't very good so I went off by myself to practice and practice to become a better player. I threw the ball at a bull's eye on our grade school building. This helped me to develop accuracy. I'd try to catch the ball and throw it back in one motion. I also practiced being on uneven ground and bouncing the ball against the wall.

In the beginning there wasn't any noticeable difference in my ability. After a lot of practice, I started to improve. My concentration was always on the ball. I don't ever remember beating Shun, but he had to work hard to beat me.

Sports were important in our family and my brothers were gifted athletes who played all sports very well. In any tough contest they moved their concentration up a couple of notches. This showed their determination and how well they could adjust to any situation.

My physical disability prevented me from achieving their level of play, but I didn't worry about something I had no control over. Even though I could not match their skills, most of the time I was able to make the play. It never occurred to me that playing baseball or any other sport was very unusual for a kid with spina bifida. God blessed me with the desire to do my best. I worked hard to be a good player and practice made a huge difference.

The kids mocked my style and made fun of my awkwardness. It was a tough time and hard for me to control my temper. Many times, I failed because of my anger. Finally, after feeling sorry for myself, desire to become a better athlete took over and I just ignored them.

Despite the terrible ridicule, playing a sport was very beneficial. I was on the field playing against stiff competition. Whenever I was able to do something productive, my focus intensified. I worked hard to do my best and had fun while doing it.

As it turned out, my playing had to be better because of my physical disability. I wasn't given many opportunities to play because a cripple was considered a loser and that is how they made me feel. Shun's encouragement always lifted my spirits. If I failed, I'd get up, knock the dirt off myself, and try again. This is how I spent most of my time.

Shun taught me to use my height to my advantage. At four eleven and a half, I could crouch down and give the pitcher a much smaller strike zone. My batting stance gave me the opportunity to hit away, chop, bunt, or try to place my hit where no one was able to catch it. If someone moved from their position, I'd try at the last minute to hit the ball through the spot the player just left. My arms were much longer than normal which made it easier to field grounders. I could also run much faster since the surgery had corrected my feet.

Shun and I were always together, joking all the time and it was fun practicing together. He took the time to explain what he was teaching me which helped me understand how to improve. Once I understood, it was easier to visualize how to make the play.

I'd watch to see how the batter held the bat. If they choked up, it could be a bunt and I'd run in on it. If the ball were chopped down, I'd run in and try to catch the ball just as it bounced off the ground. If my timing was off, the runner would be standing on first base when the ball came down.

Whenever a player beat me, I'd always say, "That was a nice play," or "You hit that well, but I'll get you the next time." If I wanted to be as good as the better players, I had to play opposite them. Winning wasn't as important to me as playing.

My most important goal was to enjoy the competition. Most people with spina bifida wouldn't even try to play sports. My problem was I wasn't smart enough to realize that. I just wanted to see what I could do.

Severe pain wasn't going to prevent me from learning how to play and enjoy the sport. If I goofed on a play, which often happened, I'd make jokes about my ability. We all had a good laugh. This released the pressure and helped me to relax.

Shun never gave in to me when playing sports. That would have made me angry. I expected him to play as tough against me as he did with others. Playing an opponent without mercy teaches an individual to improve. After learning Shun's moves, I'd wait before responding. Each time my playing improved though I was unable to beat Shun. He was an excellent player, but many times my tough playing gave him a lot of trouble.

Whenever we practiced something I would continually hear, "This is what will happen." Then we practiced what he said until it became second nature to me. Whenever I made a mistake Shun would say, "What you did took you out of position. If you had done it this way, maybe the result would have been different." When things didn't work, Shun didn't become discouraged with me. He would work me a little harder until I understood what must be done. Shun was the first one to tell me how pleased he was whenever I made positive strides.

His encouragement instilled in me the desire to always rise to the occasion. Many times it was difficult, but it was important to try. Shun taught me more than how to play different sports. He taught me to always give my best effort, all the time.

20

When Shun was invited to a party, he always included me. At one of these parties, Shun gave his coat to the host and walked into the next room. When I handed my coat to Beryl he said, "You're only here because Shun won't come unless you are invited. I sure don't want you here."

Beryl still had my coat in his hand when I quietly said, "Give me my coat. I don't want to be in a place where I'm not wanted."

"You might as well stay, now. You're here." Beryl must have thought Shun would go home if I left.

"No, I'm leaving. Give me my coat."

"Are you big enough to take it away from me?" Beryl asked.

"If you don't give me my coat, you'll find out in a hurry." Beryl gave me my coat and I went into the other room to tell Shun I was going home.

Shun asked if I wanted him to go with me. I said, "No, I'll be fine. I just don't feel like being here."

Back home Mom asked where Shun was. "He's still at the party. I didn't feel like staying." I told Mom the only reason I was invited was to make sure Shun would go.

"Shun should have come home with you."

"Is Shun supposed to look after me in everything I do? He's not responsible for me, I am."

"No, he's not responsible for you. He just enjoys your company and I like seeing the two of you together."

Years later, at a reunion, I asked Shun, "When we were growing up, did Mom tell you to keep an eye on me, or did you do that yourself?"

"No, Mom never told me to do that. I wanted you to go with me because we had so much fun together."

"I didn't think you would take me some place if you didn't want to. I'm pleased you cared enough to want me to go with you."

Another time, at a family reunion, Shun asked me, "If there was anything you could change, what would it be?"

"I'd want to give back to you all the opportunities you missed," I said. "You gave up so much to improve the quality of my life."

"Don't take that away from us. That's how we grew. Seeing you overcome your struggles and suffering inspired the family. We all wanted to help in any way we could, especially with all the pain you've had to endure."

"I've had pain all my life. I don't know what it would be like without it."

"When I would see you in such pain," Shun said, "I've often wanted to take your place, so you wouldn't have had to suffer so much."

"With the whole family behind me, I didn't feel I was going through it by myself. Your love has made a big difference in helping me maintain a positive attitude. You've always been there for me in every way. I could never quit because I'd be letting you down, when you had given me so much support. You've made my life richer beyond my wildest dreams."

Whether Shun remembers this or not, I'll never forget it. Sometimes when I'm down, I think of his love and devotion. Maybe someday, someone will look at me the way I see my beautiful brother Shun.

21

When I was about fourteen, my friend Dick's mother came into the Post Office to see my mother. We lived above the Post Office on the second floor, so Mom came upstairs after she went home and asked me if I knew Dick?

"Yes, I know him."

"Well, he told his mother he was playing football and after making a good play, you got mad and beat him up and kicked him in the hip."

"He's lying to his mother. I didn't hurt him. He watches us play sometimes, but that's it. He injured his hip about six months ago when we were sledding so he doesn't play with us much anymore."

Following this, each time I saw Dick he'd go the other way. He must have been afraid of what I was going to do to him, but I had no intention of hitting him. Dick owed me an explanation of why he had lied to his mother. When I finally caught up with him, I asked, "Why did you lie to your mother? I never hurt you. We both know that. Tell me what happened."

Dick was late getting home and his mother was angry. He had developed a slight limp following the earlier sledding accident which he hadn't told her about. For six months his limp worsened and when his mother asked him about it, he knew he was in trouble, so made something up to arouse her sympathy and avoid a spanking.

After that Dick and I remained friends. Our friendship was special and we enjoyed each other's company. We were good for each other and spent many evenings sitting on his front porch planning our futures. Our dreams were so big. We both felt there wasn't anything we couldn't do and someday people would recognize who we were.

We were thought of as cripples who wouldn't amount to anything. What we didn't realize at the time was that our lives were important. It isn't what others think of our outside appearance, what's on the inside matters. We both knew it was important to develop a positive attitude to become better kids.

Dick's hip would remain a problem for the rest of his life. The pain was so severe that the doctors had him on medication all the time.

Years later I learned Dick took an overdose and died. He didn't have many friends and probably wasn't missed by a lot of people, but the loss of our friendship was difficult for me to adjust to. I recalled his laughter and humor and had many pleasant memories of our time spent together. Losing Dick saddened me and it was a long time before I was able to talk about him.

22

I was in the fourth grade at age fourteen, when a bully in our class decided to make an example of me. At five feet ten and 180 pounds, Donny's size was intimidating. If we were standing in line to go to the bathroom, or for a drink of water, or going out to recess, he'd make his move. He would wait until the teacher was preoccupied, and then hit me as hard as he could with his body to knock me down. When the teacher would turn around to see what had happened, she would find me lying face down on the floor but did nothing about it.

My balance wasn't very good and when I hit the floor, the sudden bump sent tremors through my body and caused me to ache for days. Whenever he did one of his numbers on me, he'd wait for my painful reaction. Donny stood over me ready to hit me whenever I tried to stand up. "You're a cripple," he said. "Get out of my way!" Fighting Donny would have taken too much energy and what little I had was needed to endure my severe pain. When I didn't answer his anger intensified.

I came to school the next day in a deep black mood because of the pain. Donny started on me again the moment he saw me, shouting from twenty feet away. I'd had enough of him and told Donny to lay off me. My skin felt so hot with anger, if anyone had touched me, they would have burnt their fingers.

I started walking toward Donny and saw the fear in his eyes. No one had ever challenged him before because of his size.

I was ready for a fight, but Donny would have to start it. All of a sudden he ran toward me. He landed his first punch and before I could respond, beat me until I had no energy to defend myself.

Some of my classmates ran into the school to get the teacher. When she came out and asked who started the fight, Don pointed to me and said, "He did."

The teacher asked me, "Did you start the fight?"

"Donny has been pushing, hitting, and tripping me all year. Today I started the fight after he insulted me. If he ever starts anything again, he'll be in for the fight of his life."

"You think you took a beating today, you wait until I see you later." The teacher took both of us back into school and we were disciplined.

Knowing Donny as I did, I knew it was just a matter of time before he'd try something again. When it happened I'd be ready for him. I watched how he intimidated the kids who were afraid of him, knowing they wouldn't fight back. Donny was very slow and deliberate when he was setting a person up to hit, pushing them back with his hands, trying to knock them off balance. Donny became over-confident once he fought and won. I watched what he did and planned how to counter his moves. He had trouble moving from side to side, which would improve my chances of beating him. It was important to show the rest of the kids that Donny could be defeated.

When he decided to teach me another lesson in front of the kids, he started making comments, tripping, and jabbing at me. I continued to walk away as if I were afraid of him. Thinking I was running scared, he stood in front of me swinging at my face, but never hitting me.

Donny just wanted an excuse to hit me and my silence made him angry. "You're nothing but a cripple."

"So, since I'm a cripple, you think you can lick me. You don't have the guts to pick on someone your own size, who can fight back, do you?"

Donny wasn't going to bait me into starting the fight. He continued to swing his fist pretending he was coming after me. I put my arms up to defend myself and Donny backed off to trick me into dropping my defense. I had seen him attack others from the front so I turned my back to him and walked away. This made Donny angry and he yelled, "Don't turn your back on me."

When I stopped and turned, I saw him rushing toward me ready to swing. I saw the punch coming and ducked out of the way. "I'm not fighting you." Donny charged and swung again as I stepped to his side. He fell to the ground, embarrassed and came after me again. Whenever Donny swung, he telegraphed his punch. This gave me plenty of time to get out of his way.

Finally, I had had enough. I ducked under his swing and with all my strength punched him in the stomach. It not only knocked him down, but knocked the wind out of him as well. He doubled over with pain. My swing increased his anger and he came after me again, becoming a little crazy when he couldn't hit me.

When the teacher came out and saw Donny swinging and my stepping away to defend myself, she grabbed him and drug into the classroom for discipline.

For the next couple weeks, Donny walked away whenever he saw me. If we did come face to face, I'd speak to him with no intention of fighting.

One day when I came out of the school, I saw a lot of kids in a circle and went over to see what was going on. This big kid was picking on Donny, the way he had picked on a number of us. "Why are you picking on me?" Donny asked, "I didn't do anything to you?"

"You're a bully and I don't like bullies," the big kid answered. "I'm going to teach you a lesson."

When I heard this I said, "You're going to beat him up because you don't like bullies. What does that make you? You're doing what he has done to others. You're no better than he is." The big kid looked at me and then at Donny. He turned back and looked at me, as if I were the one who was going to take the beating. He took a step toward me then turned and walked away.

As I started for home, Donny ran up and asked, "Why did you stand up for me? No one has ever done that before. You're the last one I'd expect to do that after all I've done to you."

"Donny, I've always liked you. I didn't like your bullying."

Donny turned and walked away without a word. After a few steps, he turned back and said, "Hey Jim; thanks. I'll see you later."

The best way to turn an enemy into a friend is to stand up for him. It's difficult to do that for someone who has picked on you, but I knew that Donny was suffering so I defended him. The other kid was much bigger and I was surprised when he walked away.

I didn't feel special when I stood up for Donny. I just felt bullying was wrong and I had to try to stop it. Helping someone gave me a good feeling in my heart. It never occurred to me that this would begin a friendship that would last for years.

23

While I was in the fourth grade, a friend of our family said to me, "I bet you can't walk on your hands."

"Sure, I can,"

"If you can do it," Chuck said, "I'll buy you an ice cream cone." An ice cream cone was something very big following the Depression and the war. Very few people had money to buy any extras. I'd never done this before, but with the opportunity of having a free ice cream cone, it was worth a try even if I would fail.

I flipped up on my hands and walked about four or five steps and came back down. Chuck was as surprised as I was. "I didn't think you could do it, Jimmy." He took me into Mom's ice cream parlor and said to the others as he was buying me the cone, "You should see what Jimmy can do. He can walk on his hands. If you want to see him do it, you'll have to buy him an ice cream cone."

The people in the store didn't believe I could do this. I was offered an ice cream cone to prove it. I ate a lot of cones. The most surprising part of this was my hands and arms were strong enough to support my weight for as long as they did.

"Jimmy, don't walk on your hands unless they pay to see you do it," Chuck advised. "That way you won't have to buy any ice cream cones for a long time."

My body has always been top heavy because the spina bifida prevented my lower body from growing naturally. There wasn't much weight in my legs and my hands and arms handled the weight very easily. I found it was much easier to walk on my hands than on my feet and there was a lot less pain.

This became a way for me to earn a lot of ice cream cones and pop. I always followed Chuck's advice and never did it just to show off. People wouldn't pay for a cone if they saw me walking on my hands all the time.

At the time I started walking on my hands, my chest, shoulders, and arms were extremely big. The upper part of my body was abnormally oversized and walking on my hands strengthened my muscles. I was able to flip forward as well as backward, when I walked on my hands. Also I was able to do cartwheels with one or two hands.

The strength in my arms increased until I was able to walk a city block on my hands. This was fun exercise that increased my strength and decreased my pain.

I was unable to understand my lessons, so learning became a major problem at Bellwood Grade School. I worked very hard to complete my schoolwork. Still for some reason my accomplishments never pleased the teacher. Mrs. Ashe knew I was struggling, but always seemed impatient when I asked for help. I tried to please her and found it very frustrating when she could only find fault with me.

Even though I was dumb, I tried to improve. To show her I cared, I would help her with whatever she wanted me to do. I offered to take out the erasers and clean them for the next class.

After the wind blew the chalk dust into my face, I came back in looking like a snowy white dwarf.

Whenever something wrong happened at school, Mrs. Ashe would ask me about it. One day she had to step outside the classroom to talk to someone, which gave the kids an opportunity to go wild. I knew when she came back into the room and saw the kids running around, I'd be questioned. Thinking I couldn't be blamed for things I didn't see, I took out a book and ignored the chaos. My eyes were looking down engrossed in my reading when she finally returned. As soon as she walked in the kids headed for their seats.

She looked directly at me and asked, "What's going on in here?"

I didn't answer her and she said, "James, why are these students misbehaving?"

"I don't know," I said. "I was busy reading my book. I wasn't paying attention to what was going on."

"I'll give you three minutes to tell me who started this. If you don't tell me in that time, you'll be spanked."

"Why wait three minutes? You're wasting your time. I'm not going to tell you anything."

She waited for three minutes and asked me again, "James, what are you going to tell me?"

"I didn't do anything wrong and have nothing to say. If you're going to spank me, let's get it over with."

Her face was red with anger. She marched me out into the hall and said, "Bend over."

"I'm not bending over for you. You'll have to spank me while I'm standing up."

She gave me the spanking and said, "You'll stay in school at recess and every recess until you tell me exactly what happened."

"Well, you might as well plan on me being here for a while. I'm not telling you anything." When we returned to the classroom, I was so angry that I started slamming my books all over my desk and the floor.

"I want you to be quiet and stop throwing those books around and if you don't you'll get another spanking."

After school the kids in my class ran to my home to tell Mom what Mrs. Ashe had done to me. As soon as I walked into the house, Mom asked me what happened at school. When I told her she asked me, "Were you disrespectful?"

"I thought I was being treated unfairly and I stood up for myself."

Mom went down to see Mrs. Ashe that night after talking to me. After hearing her side of the story, Mom asked to be informed if there were any problems in the future.

It was up to me to make the most out of the rest of the year. Whenever she asked me to do something, I did exactly what she wanted it, but without enthusiasm. My anger was still strong and I knew my attitude was a problem. Whenever I saw her coming, I would walk away. I just didn't want to be around her.

Gradually, as my attitude changed toward her, my voice became softer when responding to her questions and we eventually became friends.

She invited our fourth-grade class out to her farm to see the animals and have a picnic. While at the farm Mrs. Ashe asked me to show her parents how I could walk on my hands and do cartwheels. Everyone was delighted by my performance and I was happy to be finally accepted.

24

I walked out of my fifth-grade classroom at Bellwood Grade School and saw some kids standing in front of the building, on both sides of the steps looking down on Lucy. She had a speech impediment and Dick and a few of his friends mocking her and laughing.

Dick was a bully who would not confront anyone without his gang. He would make an unkind remark and follow it with a sarcastic laugh. The other kids would join in, thinking he was funny. I had watched Dick and knew how he thought and would react. Each time he was challenged one on one, he backed down.

I walked over and stood by Lucy's side and told the kids to stop making fun of her. When Dick started to mock me, I rushed over and grabbed him by the front of his shirt.

"You lay off Lucy. You are not going to make fun of her and get away with it."

"Oh, she's your girlfriend," Dick sneered.

"You better believe it buddy," I said, "If you ever give her a hard time again, I'll be looking for you and you won't like it."

"You think you're so tough. I'm not afraid of you," he laughed.

"Go ahead, say something smart. I'll show you right now I'm not kidding."

The rest of the kids stopped teasing Lucy and Dick finally backed down after losing the support of his friends.

After the incident I asked Lucy how the kids were treating her.

"The kids won't say anything when you're around, but when you aren't, they're really mean to me."

"Do you mind if I walk you home? Maybe this will stop them. I won't get in your way or bother you."

"I'd like that, but I don't want to cause you any trouble."

"It's not a problem, Lucy. I know how painful their treatment can be."

At four eleven Lucy and I were about the same size, but she was much prettier and she looked much better in a skirt than I would have. The kids thought we looked cute together, but we were just friends.

Most of the kids still looked at me as a cripple, but Lucy never did. In the eyes of her friends, I was her boyfriend, though I wasn't smart enough to know what it meant to have a girlfriend.

Dick never failed to make some comment. One day I said to him, "Are you pleased with yourself? You must think you're pretty tough. It takes four or five of you to pick on a girl who can't defend herself. I'll tell you this, if anyone of you took the time to know Lucy, you'd find she is a very nice girl who's special." This just reinforced the idea that Lucy was my girlfriend.

We would wait for each other after school and I'd walk her home. Whenever we had school functions, we would ride the bus together. We did everything together and had a great time. The kids continually teased us about being in love.

She always dressed up which made her look like a little doll. Lucy was beautiful, besides being neat, with a gentle disposition and a great sense of humor. Lucy's gentle attitude was an inspiration to me. She had a very difficult time expressing herself. Yet her inability to speak plainly never upset her. If she rushed while talking, it became more difficult to understand her. When we were together, she took as much time as she needed to express her thoughts. She was easy for me to talk to and was very intelligent.

The kids were right in one sense. The relationship was great because we took time to share our thoughts and feelings. I really loved her but I never believed I could have a girlfriend.

I knew from watching kids who had girlfriends how restrained they were when their girls were around. Lucy and I were always at ease with each other because of our open and accepting friendship. It was nice for me to have someone to talk to who didn't ridicule me. Lucy never wanted to hurt anyone and her vulnerability made me want to protect her. The feeling of having a friend waiting for you after school, just to be with you, was very special.

If the kids knew how much their ridicule stung and the devastation of being put down, they would know what terrible feelings they caused. It was always difficult for me to understand why four or five people ridiculed one defenseless person. This made me angry.

One would start it, another added to it, someone would snicker, and more unkind remarks would follow with sarcastic laughter.

Their willingness to put someone down must have given them the feeling they were building themselves up, but they didn't stand as tall as the one they abused.

These kids were not going to get away with treating Lucy as if she were dirt under their feet. She had the ability to always say something nice, just at the right time, which uplifted the spirits of others. God blessed her in so many ways. In my eyes, Lucy was very precious.

25

Reverend Sam at the Baptist church our family attended said, God would provide you with a new body. "When we are saved and go to Heaven, we will be new creatures in Christ." While his messages were always good, this sermon in particular resounded in me.

My body ached all over with severe pain. His statement about being a new creature really touched me. Without realizing it, I stood up and said, "Will God give me a new body?" I was startled and embarrassed because I had interrupted the service. When I sat down I said, "I really hope so because the one I have really hurts."

Reverend Sam looked down at me with tears in his eyes and said, "Yes, Jimmy. You'll have a new body without any pain." I thought I would be in trouble for interrupting his service and not adding anything, but Reverend Sam's gracious response made me feel special.

This idea inspired me. The pain was so difficult to deal with and I wanted out of this terrible body. It was nice to know that when I got to Heaven, God would have a new body for me. I knew then, in my heart, that God was there for me no matter what. This was so special. Just think, a new body and it's mine, without any pain. It was hard for me to imagine having something that beautiful.

Nothing had been said in the car on the way home from church and I expected to be scolded when we arrived. To my surprise, my mother told me how much I had touched the congregation. Many people told her I brought Reverend Sam's message closer to home and they felt it was a blessing. Can you imagine that? Me making a difference in a church service! If there was a difference, only God could have done that.

26

When I was sixteen my friends and I would often meet at the Bellwood Grade School to play football. We had pick-up games and played all day. The games were always competitive, tough, and fun.

One day I was a little early and saw a friend of mine who lived next to the school about three blocks from my home. Timmy, who was mentally handicapped, was playing by himself in his backyard inside this huge fence. He was five ten and weighed about 180 pounds. He was as strong as a bull and had to be watched constantly. Timmy was feared because of his tremendous strength and no one played with him.

While I was talking to Timmy, my friend John ran up to me and said, "You better get away from Timmy. He'll hurt you."

"Timmy and I are friends," I said. "He won't hurt me."

"He's retarded and can be mean."

"Yes, he's handicapped and he'll be mean if you pick on him."

John wasn't satisfied and said, "You know that he doesn't understand what you say. If you're mean to him, he's not smart enough to know what you're saying or doing to him."

"Do you really believe that?"

"Yes, I do."

I looked at Timmy and said, "Timmy, you're my friend aren't you?" Timmy nodded in agreement.

"Did you see that?" John said. "I think he understood what you said."

"Would you hurt me Timmy?" He shook his head no. My friend did not believe what he saw.

"Aren't retarded kids stupid? It's hard for them to learn, isn't it?"

"Timmy is not stupid. He does have trouble with learning, but he usually understands what people say to him even though he doesn't speak."

"You mean he knows and understands what we say when we are around him?" John asked.

"Yes he does." I looked at John and asked, "When I talk to you, do you think I know and understand what you are saying?"

"Yes, there isn't anything wrong with you."

"Isn't that amazing? The feelings you have about Timmy are the same ones that you had for me."

"I've never felt that way about you."

"Do you remember the time when you, Ron and some of your friends chased me from the junkyard across the street and down the road? You called me names while you were hitting me with sticks and stones and made me fall. You continued this while I was lying on the ground. You treated me as if I didn't know or understand what you were saying or doing. I did know what was going on. My hearing is very good and I heard your put-downs and I understood them. I'm not that dumb to be taking a beating and not know who did it."

"Man, you remember every detail, don't you?"

"It's not hard to remember every detail because it was a nightmare. Everyone did what they wanted and didn't care about my feelings. If I showed any emotion, you'd have done something else to me. When I hit Ron with the bolt, I was so mad that I wanted to kill all of you. I tried not to stay mad, because the anger would fester like a boil and it would only hurt me. You were afraid when you saw what I did to Ron, but do you think I'd try to hurt you now?"

"No, I know you wouldn't."

"Neither would Timmy," I said. "If we're kind to him, he'll respond in the same way. Timmy is very special because that's how God made him. It doesn't matter that he's retarded because God blessed him with a beautiful spirit. If we took time to know Timmy, his spirit would have an opportunity to touch our hearts. We have to give him a chance to open up. If we do, you'll see a beautiful person whom God has really blessed."

It was as if a light went on in John's head and he realized for the first time what I was saying to him. It was important for John to give Timmy the same consideration he gave me. Sure, Timmy was retarded, but in that huge body was a heart full of love and appreciation just trying to come out. If anyone doubted it, all they had to do was become Timmy's friend. Then they could see for themselves.

Kindness was the key. I told John it was up to us to look beyond Timmy's disability and use the key to unlock his feelings.

John was surprised by the depth of my understanding of Timmy's disability. He showed his appreciation by treating me differently from that day on. Our good friendship improved when John saw a side of a handicapped person very few take the time to see.

Whenever people share their thoughts without bitterness, it helps their understanding. They make their world just a little better, especially when God is included. God did that for both of us. We said good-bye to Timmy and left to play football.

My conversation with John made a good impression and his respect for us grew. "You know Jim," John said, "you are special just like Timmy."

"Gee, thanks John." My spirit was touched. I felt the strong glow of God's blessing warming my body.

A few days later, when we were playing football at the grade school, Timmy got out of his yard. Someone had left the gate open and to Timmy, this was an invitation to see the outside world. If the gate was open, he'd leave the yard and run all over the neighborhood. No one was able to catch him because of his speed. If it were possible to stop him, no one knew how to take him home without getting hurt. Timmy fought any effort to do that.

One of the kids said, "Hey, Timmy's out of his yard. He's standing over there."

"Hey Timmy, come over here," I yelled. Timmy ran right over to where we were. I was kidding with him and started to tickle him. He responded by defending himself and tickling me. We were making a lot of noise. He was too strong for me to stop. We wrestled for quite a while. In all this time, Timmy was careful not to hurt me. I knew without a doubt he wouldn't.

The noise from our wrestling was loud enough that Timmy's father heard us. He was afraid Timmy might hurt someone. When he saw Timmy on top of me, he was really concerned and didn't understand we were playing.

I knew Timmy wasn't allowed out of the yard and this was one way for me to keep him occupied until his father came looking for him. His father was very angry and said, "Timmy, I want you to go home, now. Do you hear me?" Timmy responded by shaking his head, "Yes."

"Timmy and I were playing. I knew that he shouldn't be out of his yard. Please don't be angry with him. I'm the one who started to tickle him. It was the only way I knew to keep Timmy here with us."

"Jimmy, he could have hurt you. Don't you know that?"

"No, Timmy and I are friends. He'd never hurt me." I looked at Timmy and asked, "Aren't we friends, Timmy?" He nodded. I asked him, "Would you hurt me?" He shook his head.

Timmy knew his father didn't allow him out of the yard and he had disobeyed. I saw the fear in his eyes and was sure his father was going to discipline him.

"Please don't punish him for playing with me. It was my fault for calling him over. If you want to punish someone, punish me."

"Jimmy, you and Timmy really are friends, aren't you?"

"Yes, we are good friends. I talk to him every day when I see him in the back yard by the fence. No one else goes near him because he's different. We're both different and I wanted him to know I was his friend."

Timmy's father was very pleased that I showed that much interest in Timmy. What he didn't know was that I knew and understood what it was like to be on the outside looking in and not finding a friendly face. When Timmy looked at me, he saw a funny friendly face looking back, smiling.

I felt good helping Timmy. He trusted me and that was the best feeling. This made our friendship very special though I had trouble understanding him. It was impossible for him to put sentences together. It didn't matter because we had a communication that we both understood. We were looking for the same thing. We wanted to be judged on the inside of our heart, not our outside appearance. Love is stored in the heart. The outside is only a shell. We're more than that. If anyone takes the time to look inside, they'll see the love and understand that it is out of this world, because it comes from God.

The beauty of God's special children like Timmy is that he isn't interested in put-downs, or hurting anyone. He wants to enjoy how God has blessed his spirit with His love. This love is so pure; Timmy can't see anything but the good in others. His world is beautiful and his willingness to share it with me made my life even better.

God gives us opportunities to share our happiness and love. Special children like Timmy aren't afraid to share their love and they improve our lives. What a wonderful world this would be, if we all saw the world through their eyes.

Timmy certainly was a blessing to me and we remained friends while I attended Bellwood Grade School. Whenever I saw him at the fence, I'd go over and visit with him. We talked a lot with each other. Later when I went on to high school, I didn't see Timmy as much. Whenever he saw me he'd yell to let me know he still knew who I was.

I have no idea what attracted me to Timmy. There was no doubt that he was mentally handicapped but I wanted to be his friend. Because of his condition, he didn't have anyone to relate to. Knowing how ridicule and thoughtlessness can hurt, I was determined none of it would come from me.

If anyone picked on him while I was there, I'd defend him. Whenever anyone was mistreated, I'd make a stand for them. Isn't that what Christ did for us when He went to the cross? I am not comparing myself to Christ, I'm just trying to follow His example. We can make a difference when we stand up for those who can't stand up for themselves.

Walking with God at this early age gave me the desire to see situations through the eyes of those going through difficult times. Once I recognized their problems, if nothing could be done, I would at least give them my support and let them know I really care.

I saw no bitterness in Timmy at all. The light that sparkled in his eyes lit up my world. I wasn't doing him any favors being his friend. Friendship means sharing and caring for each other and we really cared.

27

When I was in the fifth grade, Barb started helping me with my homework. She was one of my best friends and lived in McGrann about three blocks from my home. I had always known her family and at age six I pretended to be a racecar driver next to her father's junkyard.

Barb and I were together almost all the time. During the many times my spina bifida confined me to bed, Barb brought my studies home and helped me to work through them. She had a much better understanding of the subjects than I did and spent extra time with me until I knew my schoolwork by heart. Barb's caring and concern made this a really special time.

Once after a difficult struggle doing my homework, I asked my mother, "Why am I so dumb?"

"You're not dumb," she said. "The best learning years are from birth to three. You've been in the hospital so much and have not had the same opportunity to learn as other children. Don't ever think you can't learn. Just always try to do your best. You can't ask for more than that. I have faith in you. You'll do all right because you never quit. That's why you will be successful someday."

Even with my best effort my retention was poor. I refused to be a failure and worked hard to change my image with the teachers. It wasn't so important to change their view of me as it was to change my self-image and prove to myself I wasn't a failure.

Working with Barb was a long slow process, but she had tremendous patience. To help my retention, I would reread the material and write it out and read it again. Then I would try to find a keyword to associate with the topic to remind me of the lesson. The combination of reading and writing drills and association with something familiar helped my recall. Once I had it, I didn't forget it.

I'd take my test papers home and look up the correct answers for those I missed on the test. After finding them all, I took my paper to the teacher. She checked to see if my answers were correct. When she marked some wrong, I would try again until I had the right answers for all the questions. Many times when the teacher would have given me the answer, I would say, "I won't learn unless I look it up." I did this with each test. I kept all my test papers and would study them for the semester test.

To review for a test, Barb would explain what I had learned and she was smart enough to know what might be tested. After her explanation, she would have me read and tell her what I had read. If I missed a point, Barb would have me read it over again. I had no problem reading the words. I understood what they meant. My real problem was I tired very easily and became discouraged, which made it harder to concentrate. It took me about an hour to finish each subject and be ready for class the next day.

Barb never lost interest in teaching me. Sometimes I would confuse information or events which made her laugh. This eased my tension. She continued to encourage me and never became angry with how slow I was. This always amazed me.

When we reached seventh grade, we were assigned to different classes and my retention during class was very close to zero. I'd try so hard, but my attention was often drawn out the window. It would have been impossible for me to learn had it not been for Barb's dedication to helping me after school. I was seventeen and having the most difficult time of my life. It was so bad I wanted to quit school. Barb's encouragement prevented that thought from staying in my mind very long.

Whenever I'd do well on a test, I would run over and show Barb my grade. She would be very pleased and shared my happiness. Many thought Barb was my girlfriend, but we didn't want to ruin our friendship with that kind of relationship. I just knew that I loved Barb as a very special friend. We did everything together. If anyone gave her a hard time, I'd be there to stop them.

Whenever we were not in school, Barb and I would go over to Carley's Variety store for something to eat or a milk shake and spend time with the Carleys. We shared a lot of good times with these fine people. They were interested in all of us.

Barb was so special because she brought more than her ability to teach me how to study. Barb walked me through my most difficult study problems and continued to help me understand the tests, so that the final exam would be much easier for me. She never quit in her determination to make me the very best I could be. I appreciated her willingness to spend so much time with me so that I could learn. It was especially nice to have a precious friend. She continued to help me in school until I finally graduated. I've honestly felt that I would not have graduated from high school, if it were not for Barb's dedication.

When I moved away from McGrann, there was no way I could forget Barb and her special impact on my life. She was one of the brightest spots in my often dark world. Without Barb's friendship my tremendous growth would never have happened. She was a great blessing to me. I'll never forget her devotion. She took a broken spirit and mended it with her love.

28

I wasn't allowed to play football because of my soft spot, but when I reached the fifth grade; my mother reluctantly gave me permission. Kittanning High School's junior football league had six to eight teams in the fifth- and sixth-grade league and about the same number in the seventh- and eighth-grade league. Our McGrann teams were always very good because we played football year round so our fifth- and sixth-grade team was placed in the seventh- and eighth-grade league. Whenever we played, our town's rivalry with Kittanning was on our minds.

The Kittanning High football players were the referees for our games. When Mike, Kittanning's All-State fullback, went over our lineup and saw the name Byron on our roster, he came to our bench and asked, "Which one is Jimmy Byron?" My teammates pointed to me. He came over to me and asked, "Are you Jimmy Byron?"

"Yes, I am."

"Are you any relation to Tommy Byron?"

"Yes, he's my brother."

"Boy, your brother is great football player. Are you as good as he is?"

"Oh, no. Tommy is really great. I'll never be as good as he is."

"You're right. Tommy is a good athlete."

Later in the game, there was a halfback on his way for a touchdown. I was the only one between him and the goal line. He tried to do his stutter step by faking one way and going another. As he was going through the motions, I faked one way and flew into him as he was ducking away. I hit him hard enough to knock the ball loose, causing him to fumble and I recovered the ball. The halfback was dizzy and sat out a couple of plays. Mike came up to me after the tackle and said, "Your brother Tommy would have been proud of you. That's just how he would have done it."

"Gee, thanks Mike. I appreciate that." Any time I made a good play, Mike was there to compliment me. We played the best team in the league and the score ended in a tie. Mike came up to me after the game and said, "You play football pretty well. You're a typical Byron, you don't brag. You just go out and do your job. You're pretty special, Jimmy." I felt that was high praise coming from an All-State football player.

This was the best game I'd ever played. Mike's kindness and interest in me was due to my brother Tommy and that made me feel special. It was no wonder so many people wanted to be like Mike. As well-known as he was, he was still a regular guy. That's what made him so special to all of us.

Mike didn't allow all the hype of being an All State football player go to his head, or get in the way of his being a nice guy. In my opinion, Mike was an excellent example to follow, and I did that.

It was true my brother Tommy was a great athlete. He was even greater as a person. Mike and Tommy played well against each other. Once Mike had the ball in his hands and took a couple of steps, he was like a runaway train. The only way to stop Mike was to hit him before he started to run.

"Someday, you'll be as good as Tommy," Mike told me.

"No, that isn't possible, but thanks for the compliment. It's nice of you to say that."

Mike occupied a place in my heart. The other players took notice and treated me much kinder after that.

I knew who Mike was before he singled me out. He was so popular because of his humility. After the game, I walked off the field a winner. Mike made me a better person because this huge gentle giant took the time to share his love with a little guy who didn't receive much at the time.

As I look back on this very special time, it still reminds me of a huge man whose heart was as big as his enormous body. I'll never forget his thoughtfulness toward me. It was great.

It wasn't long after this game that we met another team that was big, tough, and played smart football. These hard hitting players were well schooled in forcing the other team into making mistakes. Whenever a fumble was recovered or a pass intercepted, these players scored. They were really tough to play against. Their size as well as their excellent ability intimidated many teams.

We knew the players very well because we were friends. Each team was highly respected by the other and took nothing for granted. This was an important game because the winner would be the champion of the league.

Both sides played hard sound football. The game was scoreless until the third quarter. We moved the ball up field and then were stopped. The same happened to the opposition. As intense as the game was, the players used sportsmanlike conduct throughout the game. It was fun to play with and against such class athletes.

I was allowed to play football as long as my back and the soft spot near my tailbone were protected and I was very careful. One day, however, I ran into the opposing team's backfield to make a tackle and was blind-sided. My friend on the other team who hit me was huge. He hit my soft spot and I felt instant pain. The impact of being slammed down on the ground so hard temporarily paralyzed me from the waist down.

The person who hit me came over to me, while I was lying on the ground. "Jimmy, I didn't mean to hurt you."

"It's all right. I'm going to be okay."

"Can you move your legs?"

"No, not yet, but I will in a little while."

He stayed by my side until my brother Shun came out onto the field where I was lying. It took quite some time for my legs to come around. I lay on the ground for a long time before some of the players from both sides helped me off the field. My friend felt bad about hitting me and stayed near and I was pleased with his concern.

I lay on the sidelines for about forty-five minutes before the spasms eased and feeling returned to my legs. My back hurt like a Mack truck had just run over me.

Finally, I was able to stand. If I didn't watch how I moved, my legs would lock up at the hip and I'd fall forward. This would jar my body and be very painful, like my hip was on fire.

As my legs began to relax a little more, I walked back and forth to try to loosen them up. It still didn't do much good because my hips locked when I twisted the wrong way and caused me to fall.

After the game, we headed home, about ten miles away. Many of the players on our team took turns carrying me. I put my arms around their shoulders until they became tired and then someone else replaced them. The progress was slow and painful. We walked about five miles from the football field to the Kittanning Bridge, where we thumbed a ride home.

Shun was with me and helped steady my balance. When we finally arrived home, I tried to raise my foot to step on the landing, but my legs wouldn't move. With Shun's help, I was able to grab the banister to pull myself up the stairs. Each step felt like I was carrying a ton of weight.

Mom was in the kitchen preparing supper and heard us as soon as Shun and I started up the stairs. She looked down and saw me struggling. "You're hurt, aren't you?" Mom said.

"Yes, I'm hurt."

She had tears in her eyes and walked into the other room. She returned moments later. "Are you coming upstairs?"

"Yes, I'll be up in a little while, as soon as I can bend my knees to make the first step."

It took me a long time to climb those stairs. The pain in my back and legs was severe and took my breath away. Each step felt like someone was still hitting the soft spot in my lower back. I knew it would take days for the burning sensation to finally disappear.

In western Pennsylvania, football was the number one sport. Whenever there was a sporting event, especially a football game, the community turned out en masse for the game. Very few stayed at home unless they were sick. Even thieves must have attended the games because nothing was stolen while the games were played.

How the game was played, as well as how one acted when losing was important to the community. If anyone hurt an opposing player on purpose and was found out, the community was through with him. An individual, who played as hard when losing fifty to zero as he did when the score was tied gained a great deal of respect. To continue to try when the odds were impossible had a great influence with building character.

People in the community worked hard and they became part of the team by supporting the players. Adults would share what it was like when they played the game. This developed a lot of respect between adults and young people.

Unfortunately, these feelings were not expressed to anyone who had a mental or physical disability. For whatever reason, some people did not see how hard the disabled worked to overcome their problems. Regardless of the disability, they would make fun of a person with a handicap. If the individual did not back down against four or five people picking on him, respect would be hard won, if it were won at all. For me to gain respect, my effort had to prove to the community that whatever happened to me was accepted without complaint. It was a very slow process because my anger prevented me from standing up for myself in a positive way.

In the 1940s most adults felt a physically or mentally handicapped person should be pitied, but a handicapped person does not want pity. They want to be treated like everyone else.

The kids at school were often worse. Some of them felt my life was no more important than the dirt on the ground. Their words and actions spoke so loud it left me with a worthless feeling.

Very little was expected of any disabled person and when I played sports and did something right it was met with surprise. The general attitude was a handicapped person couldn't do anything productive because he was crippled.

God eventually taught me how to achieve success by showing me when to walk away from statements that didn't deserve an answer. Whenever I did this, my actions spoke volumes. My spiritual growth matured each time and finally, the community did sit up and take notice.

The pain would still build up in my head. The pounding sensation was so loud it felt like a drummer was playing inside my head. The beating would start out slowly and build, becoming louder and louder. It became so loud that it required all my concentration to deal with it. The severity prevented me from knowing what was going on. Again, I'd go off by myself and talk to God about what was bothering me.

My major concern was hurting someone and not knowing it happened. This was my greatest fear; that the pain would cause my mind to go blank and I'd commit an act of violence. This was another reason to go off by myself and allow the pain to leave. The only damage that occurred came when I was swinging at an object, such as a tree. I'd ask God, "In case you don't know it, this hurts. Do you know my head feels like it's going to explode?"

God would humble me with a healing balm. His spirit would fill my heart with a desire to meet the pain head on and deal with it. I'd come home with a renewed spirit and ready to tackle any problem. It was a good feeling to leave my refuge with a lot less pain. Each time this happened, God was busy developing a new attitude for me to become spiritually tough. I would face my problems, study them, work on solutions and make adjustments in my life. Little by little, He was teaching me how to do this. It was a long hard process because it was easy to take my thoughts out of God's hands and try doing it myself.

29

If my friends and I wanted to play basketball, we had to go to an orchard, about six or eight blocks from our houses. We wanted a place near home to play and there was an unused area on the Bellwood Grade School playground in McGrann. When I was sixteen, we obtained permission from the school to develop a basketball court on the playground. On the south side of the school, there was a six-inch drop-off from the regular area. It extended from one end of the playground to the other and was great for basketball because it served as out of bounds.

We measured off the basketball court. Everyone worked hard clearing the ground, using picks and shovels to break up the hard dirt. Then we pulled a chain-link fence with railroad ties across the ground to smooth out the court. We nailed the hoops and backboards to telephone poles, put them in the ground, and filled the holes tight with dirt.

With the work completed, the basketball games began. The two best players picked their teams after a coin toss. I was always chosen last. Still, when I was finally picked it made me happy to have an opportunity to play the game.

I was so bad that no one wanted me. I understood that. The constant yelling about my playing made me nervous. When someone threw the ball to me, I'd either drop it or double dribble. Either way, the other team ended up with the ball. My lack of knowledge and inability was no excuse. I was expected to play at the same level as the others. Every mistake was pointed out to me, sarcastically. I tried very hard to please my teammates, but their constant yelling made me angry. It was an impossible situation.

Whenever the ball was thrown to me and I took my eyes off it, the ball hit me in the head. If I tried to catch it I'd fumble it. I had to learn how to relax. If my eye-to-hand contact didn't improve, my plays would never become quick and smooth. The relaxation had to start in my head and work down to my hands and into my fingertips. My concentration and desire took away the self-pity. Trying to succeed made me feel good. I was going to be successful because my heart wouldn't allow me to quit.

This was the first time I'd ever had a basketball in my hands so I did whatever I was told. The captain yelled, "Bring the ball in, Jim." I tucked the ball under my arms and with great determination ran down the court with it. If anyone was in my way, I'd straight-arm them. The kids thought this was very funny. Dick was still laughing when he yelled, "You stand out of bounds and throw the ball in to one of our players."

"All you said was 'bring the ball in,' you didn't say how."

This was my first mistake. As the game continued, I made many more and Dick patience disappeared. Our tempers rose with each error I made.

"How stupid can you get?" Dick asked. "You know better than that."

"You're the one who's stupid. You didn't tell me what I was supposed to do. I don't know any better than that, because this is the first time I've ever played this dumb game. If you want me to help the team, you have to tell me what to do. And don't call me stupid."

"Yeah," Dick said, "and what are you going to do about it?"

"Well stupid, it's your move."

"Don't call me stupid again."

"I won't call you stupid again," I answered. "I'll just call you stupid."

The kids snickered and Dick replied, "Don't call me stupid."

"It's all right for you to call me stupid? And I can't say the same to you."

"I'm different than you," Dick said.

"No, we're not different. I have feelings the same as you do."

"Okay, say it again, and I'll knock your block off."

"It's your move. Once you make yours, I'll make mine. There will be two hits. One, I'll hit you and you'll hit the ground. If you're stupid enough to get up, there will be two more." He looked at me and turned away. I'm happy he did because he probably would have knocked me into the next county.

We were down at our end of the court trying to score a basket. I was standing off to one side by myself watching how the others played. I didn't know what to do. Dick asked, "What are you doing? You're to keep your man out of this place."

"I'm watching to see how the game is played," I answered.

Dick was really angry and said, "Get out of here before you get hurt."

"Do you think you're big enough to do it?" I yelled.

"Everyone is bigger than you," Dick laughed.

"Yeah, you're right, but you aren't big enough to move me." I wanted to hit someone, even if it cost me a beating. I'd get rid of this worthless feeling that weighed heavy on my heart. I had had enough of this arguing and decided to call it quits.

Walking home I decided I was going to improve, just to show myself I could do it. The continual yelling from the kids made me nervous and the constant pressure to apply myself always caused me to mess up. If ways to mess up hadn't been invented, given a minute, I'd find them.

Back home I shared the story with Mom about tucking the basketball under my arms and running down the court with it. Mom was tickled with my description and laughed. I said in a very deep voice, "It ain't funny, Mom." I told her about the abuse and how terrible it was.

"Jimmy, why don't you listen to what's said? If you need to change, work on it. If you don't, forget it. If their comments make you angry, use the anger to improve yourself. The more you become angry, the harder you must try. Just concentrate on using your anger. Allow the anger to fuel your desire and strengthen your determination. Don't allow the kids to see your anger, or know how you feel. Use your determination to become a better player or at least a smarter one. Watch what the other kids do and see how you can use what you learn to improve your ability. It's up to you to rise above it, Jimmy, if you want to become successful. This is one way to do it."

I had heard this a hundred times. Maybe it was time to listen to Mom's suggestions. On my way out I held up my basketball.

"I'm going over to the railroad tracks and learn how to dribble this blasted thing."

"You be careful on the tracks. If you see or hear a train coming, get off the tracks right away."

I had seen an ad for a Harlem Globetrotters' game on what in 1947 was the towns only TV set. Marcus Haynes had the best dribble I'd ever seen. No matter how hard anyone tried, it was impossible to take the ball away from Marcus. He was the greatest.

I thought about Mom's advice to use what I had. Just like the principles Shun had taught me when we played baseball, my own characteristics could be adapted to basketball. My body was very short, but my arms were long. Maybe it was possible to use this to my advantage. It was worth a try.

There was a fifteen-foot gully on both sides of the tracks. The tracks were higher than the river and served as a dike when the floods came. If the tracks hadn't been higher, McGrann would have flooded every spring. Though it came close many times, the water never went over the tracks.

The first time I dribbled the ball it hit a stone and shot down into the gully. I picked it up and did the same thing all over again. I spent more time going down into the gully to pick up the basketball than I did dribbling it. I'd go down the gully, pick up the ball, climb back up the steep incline, go back to the tracks, and start all over again. This continued for a couple of weeks. I tried to position myself to block the ball and prevent it from going back down into the gully. The only problem was the ball was smarter than I was. Regardless of what side I was on, the ball went down the other side.

Some of the kids I played with thought I was a little crazy because of my technique. If they had heard me talking to the basketball, they would have been convinced. My anger became so intense that I was having trouble seeing the ball. Finally, I thought of Mom's idea of trying to relax. As soon as I relaxed, the pressure seemed to come off my shoulders. Each time the ball bounced down the gully, it made me angry, but I would watch to see where my hands were when the ball shot off the tracks. I'd work a little harder and after the second week I was able to control the ball for about two or three dribbles. There always seemed to be enough success to fuel my desire and my ball handling improved each week. I was determined to be good at it no matter how long it took.

After a while it became a game. I thought of the ball as the other player. It was me against the ball. The ball would win a few rounds, but it wouldn't win the overall game. My desire didn't allow my temper to get in the way of learning how to dribble. My progress increased each week, but I still had the problem of looking at my hands while dribbling. I felt success would come when I had total fingertip control of the ball. By the fourth or fifth week my fingertips controlled the ball wherever it bounced, regardless of the ties, tracks, or stones. I was beginning to learn how to handle a basketball that didn't want to be handled.

After learning how to dribble, I had to develop the skill to control the ball with both hands. I wasn't going to allow my right hand to do all the dribbling. I spent a long time fumbling the ball

all over the place until I could include my left hand. Finally, I was able to dribble the ball on anything and control it with both hands without watching the ball.

This major accomplishment gave me tremendous confidence. I learned that all I needed to do was examine the problem, find the solution, and work toward making myself better. It was a great feeling. Wherever the ball bounced, my fingers had control of it. I could dribble anywhere, at any speed, and the ball could not get away from me. I could throw the ball from my dribbling position, with no indication that I was going to pass the ball. My small stature also made the trajectory low enough that if anyone stepped in front of the ball, it would bounce off his knees. The passes were thrown soft, without stinging the players' hands, and just out of reach of our opponents. I was able to dribble through, or behind my legs, on either side of my body. The ball was kept low enough so that no one could take it away from me.

This new confidence helped me to relax and improve. I looked back at my mistakes and found solutions so I wouldn't repeat them. This process helped me make fewer and fewer mistakes. The games were played hard and it was always important to do your best. If you lagged behind and did not play your best, you learned in a hurry that someone new would come in to replace you.

Early in my life I saw any correction as ridicule. Dealing with constructive criticism was something new and different. Whenever criticism came my way, I learned to examine it and change where needed.

I still played in the games and showed slight improvement, but not much compared to all the work I had done. No one had seen my new dribbling ability. At this point, I still didn't have the confidence to show what I had learned.

As my confidence grew my ball handling improved a little more with each game, but not quickly enough to satisfy Dick. I still had a lot to learn about the game and Dick was always angry when I didn't follow his directions. He told me again how stupid I was and that I'd never be a basketball player. Finally, I had enough of his lip and told him I was a better player than he was.

"I'll play you a game of one-on-one," Dick said.

"Are you sure you want to do this?" I asked.

We decided whoever reached ten baskets first would be the winner and the loser would buy the winner a coke. With hesitation I checked my pockets. I had a dime and since cokes were five cents each, I could afford to play at least two games.

"Are you afraid you'll lose?" he asked.

"Let's play. It's your money."

He laughed and looked at me with a smirk. "You think you can beat me, don't you? You gotta to be kidding."

"Talk's cheap. Let's see what you can do."

"I'll take the ball out first." He did and as he started to drive toward me for the score, I let him go past. I reached around the front of his knees and tapped the ball away from his hands without touching him. He was dribbling air and I was dribbling the ball. "You just made a lucky play," he said. I didn't respond, but the guys on the sidelines really enjoyed the play. He looked around and watched me dribbling the ball. I started to drive toward the basket. Dick kneed me in the thigh, knocking me out of bounds. He picked up the ball and said, "You went out of bounds; it's my ball."

"No, you pushed me out. It's still my ball."

One of the kids said, "Dick, you pushed him out of bounds; the ball belongs to Jim."

I started to drive toward the basket again and Dick did the same thing. "Do you want to fight, or do you want to play basketball?" I asked him. "I'm not going to buy you a coke if you're going to knee me out of bounds every time I drive in for a basket."

Dick grabbed the ball out of my hands and said, "It's my ball, you went out of bounds."

The same kid on the sidelines told him, "Dick, you'll forfeit the game if you don't give Jim the ball. You will have to buy the coke." Dick gave me the ball. He did whatever he could to beat me. He pushed, shoved, bumped, hit, hacked, and stepped on my feet. Finally I had enough, so I swatted at the ball and missed, smacking Dick on the side of the head. You could hear the smack all over the school ground. I said to Dick, "The foul's on me, it's your ball."

Dick did not score. Every time he brought the ball in, I'd take it away from him. He spent so much time looking for me that he forgot about scoring. Dick was much bigger, heavier, stronger and slower. When he made a move, you knew in advance what he was going to do. It was easy to defend against him. The problem with Dick was he would challenge you only if he felt he could beat you. He was a bully and I couldn't allow him to push me around. If he could bully me, he wouldn't stop. Dick would take every advantage he could.

My belting him on the head gave him a message to play the game or forfeit. Every time he became too reckless I'd pop him on the side of the head and say, "Oops, it's your ball, I fouled you." He would take the ball out, dribble a couple of times and I would take it away from him. I won the first game and Dick said, "You were lucky, let's play again, double or nothing." I checked to see if the dime was still in my pocket. It was. We played again with the same result. Now Dick owed me two cokes. This was a lot of money at that time and I was having a ball. We played again and Dick owed me four cokes.

Later on the kids asked me, "Did Dick ever pay you the cokes he owes you?"

"No. Not yet."

"Have you played him again?"

"No, I'm not playing him, until he pays me."

Dick would try to have a pickup game with the other kids. When he would offer the winner a coke, they replied, "You didn't pay Jim his cokes yet. No, I'm not playing you until you do." Well Dick didn't like me at all at this point. When the other kids refused to play him until he paid for the cokes, it made him dislike me even more. Dick felt I was the one who put them up to it. He never bought the cokes and I didn't play him one-on-one again.

Dick always felt uncomfortable around me because of the questions about the cokes. He always told me that I'd never be as good a player as he was. I was chicken because he didn't have the opportunity to win back his cokes.

For about a month Dick remained angry with me. I told him, "Don't mess with me, or I'll belt you one." The kids continued to tease him and kept his attention away from me. While Dick was distracted, I walked up behind him, took off my belt and said, "I told you, Dick, I'd belt you one." Then Dick started to laugh. The easiest way to get rid of an enemy is to make him your friend.

30

Around age seventeen, my severe back problems worsened. The soft spot on my back had become increasingly painful. Since Dr. Winters was out of town, Mom called Dr. Fichthorne whose office was about three blocks from our home. I knew Dr. Fichthorne very well because I played sports with two of his sons, Jim and Bill.

Dr. Fichthorne and I had been friends for a long time. Whenever I went to their house, he asked me how I was doing. Many times the going was rough and he encouraged me. He would say, "Jimmy, if anyone can beat this thing, you can." Our friendship was very special and enjoyable for both of us. Whenever he saw me he would stop to say hello. That thoughtfulness meant a great deal to me and gave me such a special feeling. Dr. Fichthorne treated me like a son. I loved this beautiful doctor for being my friend.

Even though I had known him for a long time, this was his first opportunity to examine me. "You're okay, Jimmy," Dr. Fichthorne said after his examination. "With all your back problems and the possibility of becoming temporarily paralyzed, I can't believe you are as tough as my sons' say you are. Jimmy, how can that be?"

"You're right, I do have a lot of back problems, but I'm not as tough as your son thinks I am. When we play football, I hit them as hard as I can with bone-jarring tackles and try to make it sting. I have to play at their level for them to accept me."

"My sons say, 'no one tackles harder than Jim Byron.' They are almost twice your size and yet you can still stop them. No matter what happens, you don't complain about your pain. You come back with such drive; my sons feel they can't beat you. They have great respect for you."

"Well, that could be for only one reason. I have a lot of respect for them as well, and besides, I'm their friend."

A few days later some of us went out to the doctor's farm about a mile out of McGrann. Dr. Fichthorne's sons put up a hoop inside the barn so we could play basketball in the winter.

When Dr. Fichthorne saw me there with the other kids he asked, "Jimmy, would you like to see what we have here on our farm?"

"Yes, I'd like that," I said. He took me all around and explained his hobby. He was growing hybrid plants and seeing increased yields. I asked him many questions and he seemed to appreciate my interest. We must have been gone at least an hour and I didn't want the tour to end.

After it was over, he thanked me for going with him. "I've wanted to show this to someone who would appreciate what I am doing here. Jimmy, you've made my day."

I told Dr. Fichthorne what a special treat this was for me. "This is the first time anyone explained what farming is all about. Yet, with your busy schedule, you took the time and showed me so much. It was great and I appreciate how nice you've been to me."

My life was only one of the many that this good doctor touched. I know I'm a better person for having been around him. My memories of Dr. Fichthorne's love warm my heart and remind me how the Lord will send an angel to comfort us in times of pain. God uses this time to prepare us for the Heavenly rewards He has for us.

31

Six weeks before going into the seventh grade, Dr. Winters talked with my mother about a new appliance that had been developed to deal with bladder problems. I'd been wearing diapers since the third grade and this new appliance would be an improvement. The lighter appliance was easier to wear and more comfortable than diapers. It was made out of hard rubber, which wore like iron and would not break or crack from the urine.

Dr. Winters felt that six weeks would give me enough time to get used to wearing it and make any adjustments before school started. Despite this long and difficult period, the appliance would allow me to begin a better life.

The appliance's pouch and bag attached to a belt in the front. The belt's two metal eyelets, an inch and a half from the hips in the front and back secured the straps. After anchoring the straps in the back eyelets the straps had to be pulled under the legs and up the front on the inside, threaded through the front eyelets by the hips and then secured. The bag was attached to the leg, with a rubber strap that wrapped around the leg. It could be set at either the side of the leg or under the knee. I tucked the bag under my knee to make the bulge less noticeable. With the penis inserted into the pouch, discharged urine drained into the attached bag.

If the pouch wasn't strapped securely enough, it leaked. The leakage could occur during vigorous activity or even while I was just sitting. The pouch always had some residual urine and sometimes when I sat down, the residue leaked from the opening. When I played sports it was important to empty the bag first. Running could stretch the straps and allow air to enter the bag through the pouch. The increasing air pressure could eventually cause the bag to pull away from the pouch. If the thin flexible bag became fully disconnected, it rested on my calf upside down and the urine leaked all over my pants.

If the urinal was strapped tightly, it prevented the urinal from leaking, but the straps shut off my circulation and caused my buttocks, hips, and thighs to have muscle spasms. If it wasn't possible for me to go to the rest room to release some of the pressure, the pain became so severe that just adjusting the straps was painful.

I found the best time to adjust the straps was a few minutes before leaving for school, but I was never able to apply the right pressure to the straps. It was always a choice between pain and leakage. Even though the pain and numbness were severe, the embarrassment of being wet was far more difficult to endure.

Whenever I'd release the straps, the blood supply came into my muscles with a force that shot fire from my hips all the way down my legs. When this happened my legs shook and the severe pain brought tears to my eyes.

Enduring the pain took so much energy and concentration that there was no room to think about other problems. I shared so much of my hurt with God and His love provided a warm feeling in my heart. This gave me the courage to continue the struggle.

My frequent failures fueled my desire not to quit and led to my many successes.

Throughout my life pain has always been severe, especially when walking. I learned to use pain as a friend rather than an enemy. Pain taught me when to back off and not to push too hard, giving my body a chance to heal. It became the enemy when I didn't pay attention to the warnings.

I always thought it was important to think about being tougher than my current crisis. When I responded to the pain with anger, I turned to prayer. After a while things became easier. Coping with my devastating situation made me spiritually stronger and I was able to control my temper. It didn't happen all at once, but I recognized the destructive nature of my anger and channeled that energy into becoming a kinder person. This was how God allowed me to live with the pain and grow.

The first time I wore the urinal to school one of my most embarrassing moments occurred in Mrs. McCoy's English class. Whenever I voided into the urinal, not all of the urine emptied into the bag attached to my leg. It was difficult to sit while wearing it and there was always the danger of urine leaking all over me and on the floor.

When this actually happened during the first week of school, I raised my hand. "May I be excused to see Mr. Miller?" Mrs. McCoy saw the wet floor and excused me. I went to the principal's office and explained to him what had happened. Mr. Miller and I were great friends. He was very understanding and allowed me to go home to change clothes. As I was leaving he said, "I'll see you in a little while, Jimmy."

"I probably won't be back," I answered feeling so empty inside from the embarrassment. I rode my bike home and walked into the Post Office below our apartment where my mother worked. Since it was unusual for me to come home this early, she looked very worried and asked what had happened.

After explaining the situation I said, "I'm not going back to school."

"If you don't want to go back to school, it's okay with me."

"I'm going to quit school," I said with tears in my eyes. My friends were all there and I really didn't want to quit.

"That's up to you. Nothing will change my feelings toward you." She smiled at me and I no longer felt alone. "Will you do something for me before you decide to quit?"

I knew what she was going to say; she had said it so often. Mom was always supportive and would encourage me to fight for my future. "Will you go back to school tomorrow and try it just one more time?"

With a heavy heart and broken spirit, I wondered if I'd be able to pick myself up off the ground. This was the lowest I'd ever felt.

"Well . . . Okay, Mom. But I'll never get over the embarrassment. Tomorrow will be the toughest day of my life. Still, I'll do it for you." I knew it had to be done. I couldn't just quit. No matter how bad it was I had to try. I would be ready for the kids and their worst treatment. Mom taught me the way to beat any situation was to pray for strength and meet it head on and that's exactly what I would do.

The next day I walked into my classroom and waited for the ridicule to start. With great fear, I tried to sneak to my seat without anyone seeing me, but the kids paid very little attention. I was surprised and pleased by the absence of ridicule and I didn't know if the students even knew what happened yesterday. I felt this was a blessing from God.

This experience encouraged me to continue in school. It made a tremendous difference in my life, showing me how to work through my problems. With God's help nothing would stop me from graduating someday.

When I came home from school, I found Mom waiting anxiously to see how my day had gone. I told her no one said anything. Once again, Mom's wisdom helped me make the right decision. She was always there for me.

32

Mr. Davis, our football coach was very interested in his players. If a player had a problem, he would call them in to see if he could help them. He was a good Christian and it showed in his actions toward the players. Coach Davis was a friend to many of the parents and he knew what was going on with his players. He was loved by everyone.

We became good friends because of his relationship with my family. Three of my brothers played on his team and he always asked my mother how I was doing. During my last year of junior high, Coach Davis talked to my mother about my becoming a football manager. He knew Dr. Winters wouldn't allow me to play football because of the soft spot on my back, but being a manager would keep me close to the team. His interest in my well-being was very special.

When I saw Coach Davis walking across the high school gym one day I said to him, "Hey Coach, I'll be out for football next year."

"Jimmy, I could really use a manager next year, would you be interested?"

"No way, those guys are treated like dirt and no one is going to treat me that way."

"Do you think that I'd treat you that way?"

"No, I know you wouldn't, but some of the players might."

"If you become my manager, I'll teach you not only to be a good one, you'll be the best."

"I'd rather play football, but I'll think about it." It never occurred to me that Coach Davis was worried about the soft spot on my back. He knew that if it were bumped, it could cause me to be paralyzed from the waist down. All I could think of was playing and how great my brothers were. My ability wasn't even close to what they had, but I'd make up for it with my hustle and determination.

Not long after that I had some back problems. Each time my back hurt, I'd go and see Dr. Winters about it. While I was in for the examination, I asked him, "May I play football next year?" Dr. Winters wasn't expecting my question so soon, but he knew it was coming because my mother told him I wanted to play.

I was lying on the examination table and he busied himself behind me. Finally he looked at me and said, "No Jimmy, you can't play."

I was totally shocked and disappointed. I looked at him and asked, "Why Dr. Winters? I've been looking forward to playing football."

With my exam completed, he guided me from the table to a chair.

"Jimmy, I would love to see you play football. But if you do and that soft spot is hit, it could paralyze you. Not temporarily but permanently."

As I sat in the chair with my head down and my spirits dragging on the floor, I thought to myself, "This darn back will never let me do anything. I'll never be anything but a cripple.

What good am I?" Spina bifida won again. The old self-pity returned and entered my heart.

"You could be a manager," Dr. Winters suggested, "and still be part of the team."

I was so disappointed that I couldn't bring myself to look at the doctor. Finally, when I looked up at him, he had tears in his eyes. I could see the hurt he felt for me. It was the first time I saw how much this beautiful doctor loved me.

Dr. Winters would have given anything to say, "Yes Jimmy, you can play." I wanted to hug Dr. Winters, to let him know I loved him too, but I was too big for that. How wrong I was. Many times I wished I could relive that moment and give him the hug.

I couldn't stop thinking about Dr. Winters' compassion and how badly he hurt for me. His sad expression really touched my heart. The more I thought about my mother's support and how Dr. Winters and Coach Davis showed an interested in me, the better I felt. God's love uplifted my spirit through them to help turn my life around once again. I thanked God for sending these beautiful people to my rescue. Their love made me feel my life was special, that I was worth something. Wow! Do you know how wonderful that feeling is?

I still wanted to play football and the decision to be a manager was difficult. If I decided to do it, I could be around the team and that was very important to me. At this point, I didn't know what I would do.

The day after I saw Dr. Winters, Coach Davis said he wanted to see me in his office. When I went in, he said, "Jimmy, I want you to be my manager. Will you?"

"Gee Coach, I don't know."

"Jimmy, why don't you give it some thought? Talk to your mother about it." He didn't push me and I told him I would.

That night at supper I told Mom what Coach Davis had said. "Are you going to do it?" she asked.

"That's hard to say. If I'm a manager, I'm going to be the very best." After we talked about it and she encouraged me, I finally decided to do it. Mom seemed pleased.

The next day, I went to see Coach Davis and said, "I'll be your football manager. I would like to take care of the players' needs so all they have to do is concentrate on the game. I want to learn how to fix broken equipment. Whatever needs to be done, I want to learn how to do it. I want to make a list of things to do before the game, so I can check them off. That way, there will be no surprises."

"You really have given this some thought, haven't you?" Coach Davis was really pleased and said, "We'll teach you everything we do."

No one knew how important it was for me to be accepted by the players than Coach Davis. He knew how much I wanted to be a part of the team and saw to it that the players appreciated what I was doing.

Joe Frick, our equipment manager, taught me how to repair equipment. Joe was pleased with my progress and proud of my accomplishments. He was so nice to me and we had a lot of fun.

Joe showed great patience and made me feel relaxed. He was a very special friend.

At this point I took my first positive step to become a productive human being. How could I ever be a failure with support from such wonderful people? My life has been blessed in so many ways.

During my third year as football manager, the Ford City High School football team was not very big, but they were quick and agile. Late in the third quarter of a scoreless game with Tarentum on their home field, Bob, our halfback ran along the sideline, was tackled and pushed out of bounds.

Our players on the bench yelled, "Look out! He's out of bounds." Bob and three others landed on top of me, just as I started to move out of the way. My soft spot hit the edge of the bench so hard that it felt like a knife had gone through my back and came out my stomach. I couldn't move my legs and told the other managers I was hurt.

I still do not understand why the coach did not see what had happened to me, or why the four other managers did nothing to help me or even tell the coach.

After the game was over, I was left alone on the field. Everyone else returned to the locker room. So I used my two heavy duffel bags filled with equipment to help me walk. I'd place one in front of me, take a step, move the other bag and take another step. The distance from our bench to the locker room was short and finally I reached the door.

Lifting my right foot to the step, my back and leg muscles contracted in a spasm so severe that all feeling left my legs and I fell backward to the ground. The coach ran out of the locker room when he heard my scream. Some players, who followed the coach lifted me very gently and carried me into the locker room, where first aid efforts were fruitless. Finally, an hour and a half after my injury, the coach realized how seriously I was hurt and an ambulance took me to the hospital.

My brother Shun, still in his football uniform, went with me to the hospital. He encouraged me to relax whenever the pain intensified. The thought of never walking again was terrifying and I thank God Shun was there with me.

More than anything else, I needed God's strength to deal with my pain and fear. I have always tried to learn from my experiences. Sometimes past mistakes can be avoided in the future, but when accidents and misfortunes are beyond my control, I just have to forget them and accept God's will. Thanking Him for all things gives me a positive attitude and I've always come away with a special blessing.

I was in the hospital for three days and when my doctor allowed me to return to work three weeks later, the players were happy to see me. It was a good feeling to return, though the spasms in my back and legs did not allow me to stand very long.

This ability to endure hardships impressed my friends and our relationships deepened. These guys who seemed so unconcerned when I was injured, now responded with kindness when they saw the change in me. My anger with my circumstances was gone and I'd thank God for His blessings regardless of the pain involved.

33

When I was twenty-two, the draft board instructed me to report to their office in Kittanning for a screening, after which we would be sent to Pittsburgh for a physical. Many of my friends said that, since I was under five feet tall, the Army probably won't take me. Most of my time had been spent around home and I wasn't looking forward to going into the service. The idea of leaving home was very frightening.

At the draft board, I filled out a number of forms about my personal history. Then an interviewer asked about my physical abilities, if I was able to march and hike. Finally, he asked me, "Do you have any physical disabilities?"

"Yes, I have spina bifida in my lower back. It was repaired through surgery."

"Does this prevent you from running, lifting, or marching?"

"I'm not allowed to do any heavy lifting, but I can run and hike."

"Do you have any other problems?" he asked.

I told him about my problems with bladder control.

"You're not five feet tall and with all your medical problems, I don't think the Army is for you."

"If I'm sent into the Army, I'll make the most of it. It may take me a little while, but I'll do as much or more than the next guy. I'm not afraid to try the service, but I don't want you to get in trouble because you let me stay behind."

He said he decided who should go to Pittsburgh for a physical. "There is no reason to send you there. They'll only send you back. It would be a waste of your time and the Army's. You can go home."

This really surprised me. Despite my condition, I thought I would be drafted. Being sent home was a relief.

He was very kind and said, "We could really use your attitude in the Army; but no, it would be too difficult for you. Your body could not handle the punishment."

My mother was surprised to see me walk into the house and tell her I wouldn't be going into the service. Many times over the years, I've wondered what kind of person I would have been, had I been able to serve in the military.

Following my army screening, I attended Pennsylvania Rehab School for a year, worked in a body shop and a trucking company. Finally I got a job at Wheaton College, where my brother Tommy graduated. Traveling out to Wheaton, Illinois was a new experience. I would stop to eat something, purchase gas, check the oil, and continue on my way. It was a good feeling to be on my own and make my own decisions. I was thinking about this new opportunity, but felt a little uneasy about what my future held.

Driving gave me a lot of time to think about some of the hatefulness and ignorance I was leaving behind. My mother was the postmaster and once when a lady came in to pick up her mail asked Mom, what sin she had committed that caused me to be crippled. She also told my mother that people like me should be placed in an institution.

My mother knew how to handle most situations. One day she told me to take the woman's mail to her. It was raining pretty hard when I got to her house and knocked. When she answered the door, I said, "My mother asked me to deliver your mail to you. She didn't want you to get wet."

"Thank you, Jimmy," she said, "I appreciate that."

A couple days later, she saw me playing with some friends and called me to come over to her house. I went in and she gave me a glass of milk with fresh-baked cookies. I thanked her and told her how much I appreciated her thoughtfulness.

The next day when she went to the post office, she told my mother what a gentleman I was. Each time she saw me, she had some cookies for me. She never again told my mother I should be in an institution. Again, Mom's wisdom made a difference. The woman's change of attitude turned out to be such a blessing to me.

My future was uncertain to everyone, even my friends. They didn't think I would succeed if I left home. If I stayed and something happened to my mother, I'd be on my own anyway. I knew I had a good place to live that didn't cost me much. I was living with my mother and my life was easy. Despite the pressure of living on my own, I wanted the freedoms and responsibilities of an adult. Still questions plagued me. What if I fail? Will I come back home a failure?

I just had to make it. No matter what the problem, I'd learn to adjust. I knew there would be setbacks, but my determination would carry me through. If I failed along the way, I'd get up and try again. In the end I would succeed because I would not quit trying.

While living in Pennsylvania, I worked with the youth group at our church and wanted to continue this in Wheaton. When my mother and I found a room for me to rent, I asked the landlady about local churches. She invited me to attend the Evangelical Free Church when I returned. She said the church had a very good youth group and they were looking for some help. She referred me to Mr. Lebo who was in charge of the program. In the meantime, she would contact him and tell him about my interest.

By the time I arrived in Wheaton and unpacked my clothes, I was sure this was the right move. My landlady invited me to join her and her son at the Alumni Gym at Wheaton College to watch a film on missionary work. I went with them and after the film was introduced to Illa Lebo.

"This is George Lebo's daughter," my landlady said. "Mr. Lebo's going to talk to you about working with young people."

Illa said it was nice to meet me. It was nice to meet her too. She was slender and nicely dressed, with shoulder-length brown hair. I thought she looked like a model. She seemed genuinely interested in me and was very kind. Under normal circumstances a man would have fallen for a girl like this, but I always thought I wasn't normal. I had been led to believe I shouldn't form romantic relationships and that I could never have a wife and family.

On our way home from the church, I told my landlady how nice I thought Illa was. "She is very nice and is like that to everyone. She's highly thought of." I would have thought more about her too, were it not for how I looked. No one would ever be interested in me. I was told this many times throughout my life. Now it was time to forget and move on.

When I reported to the college, I learned I would be working in the Admissions Office for a couple of weeks until the football coach arrived on campus. People at the college introduced me as Tom Byron's brother and everyone accepted me right away. I didn't realize it at first, but Tom had opened the way for me. He was well loved and I was proud to be introduced as his brother.

When I came to Wheaton, I understood my position would be equipment manager for all teams. My new boss, Coach Chrouser had been in Honey Rock, Wisconsin about fifty miles south of the Canadian border, where Wheaton College taught camping techniques over the summer. He came home the first week in August and my office supervisor told me to go to his home on Saturday to meet him.

So on Saturday morning I went to his house. I told him my name was Jim Byron and that the Admissions Office sent me over to meet him.

"If I wanted to meet you, I'd have scheduled an appointment in the gym." He slammed the door in my face and left me standing on the porch.

"I'm not working for a bear that treats me that way," I said to myself. My anger was so strong for the rest of the weekend that I wanted to pack my suitcase and head back to Pennsylvania, but first I had to confront the coach.

When I saw him on Monday, I was still angry and planned to tell him I was going back home. No one was going to treat me that way and get away with it.

Just before I walked in for my interview with him, I overheard one of his staff members ask, "How is your son?"

"Danny has a concussion. He's still in critical condition, but it looks like he'll come out of it."

When I heard this, I decided not to say anything about how he had treated me. I thought he might not have been angry with me, but just concerned for his son and I had been taught always to give people the benefit of the doubt.

To my surprise the coach was still angry with me for coming over to his house and told me not to do it again. I answered, "The front office told me to go over to see you. Should I have refused? If I did that I'd have been out the door and someone else would have this job."

He just stared at me as though my answer surprised him. I figured I was going to be fired anyway, so there was no reason to back down.

"I don't think that you can do the job," he said. "You don't look strong enough."

"It sounds like you've already made up your mind. You mean you're not going to hire me?"

"I need someone who will do what I say, and just the way I want it. I don't think you can do that."

"How would you know, if you don't try me out?"

"You don't look like you can do the job."

I was angry and felt my trip to Wheaton was a waste of time. If I didn't have the job anyway, he would at least know how I felt. "You're basing your judgment on my physical disability."

"All I'm interested in is your ability to do the job."

"You're not going to hire me, are you?" I asked again.

"No, I don't think so."

"You mean I've come all the way out to Wheaton, to be turned down by you because I don't look like I can do the job. You've made us both losers."

This really made him angry. "I've never been a loser in my life."

"You are now."

"How am I a loser?"

"You're a loser because you don't have the guts to give me an opportunity to show you what I can do. And I'm a loser because I can't show you what I'm able to do. My size and looks have nothing to do with it."

I had been told how aggressive he was and not to be afraid of him. Other coaches and office staff warned me and advised me not to back down. Coach Chrouser didn't like losing at anything and my suggestion that he was a loser got to him. A surprised grin, almost a defiant smile, emerged.

Coach Chrouser gave me six months to see if I could do the job. The Centennial Gym was still under construction, so I was sent to work in the front office for a few weeks. When the equipment room, called "the cage," was completed, Coach Chrouser reassigned me there. In the beginning, I thought he was very rough on me, but the man he didn't think could do the job would still be working there nearly six years later.

34

Working with the church youth group gave me the opportunity to get to know Illa Lebo better. We worked together as counselors for the fourth- and fifth-graders. Illa taught the girls and I worked with the boys.

Mr. Lebo met with his teaching staff each Sunday evening at 6:00 P.M. for half an hour before our classes. Then we were turned loose on our students, teaching the books of the Bible and how to find different passages. The girls felt that Illa was someone very special because of her devotion to them. The young people had a great time and were eager learners.

After our instruction, we went back to the fellowship hall for the Bible challenge. With the boys on one side of the room and the girls on the other, the competition began. One of the counselors for each age group would lead the contests. A Bible verse was given and the young people had to wait until the command "charge" was issued before they could begin their search. Though it seldom happened, any one starting before the command was disqualified for that verse.

When contestants found the verse, they raised their hands and the counselor called on the person to read the verse to make sure it was right. If it was incorrect the counselor called on the next person. The other counselor for each age group kept score on the chalkboard and the winning team would receive a larger share of the candy prizes. Each week, Illa and I would take turns bringing the candy. The girls beat the boys most of the time. The rivalry and teasing was all in fun and the young people learned a great deal from this training.

One week when I lead the "charge" and brought the candy, Illa's girls really beat my boys badly. After the contest I handed out the tootsie rolls to the winners. When I came to Illa I said, "Here's three more. You're too thin and we need to fatten you up." The girls laughed and after the meeting, Illa told me the girls thought I was flirting with her. Though I denied the flirtation, I told Illa how special she was and how the girls looked up to her. Sadly, I still believed I could never have a relationship. A few months later I started to rethink this belief.

The Lebos spent Christmas in Crystal Lake, Florida with their son George. I was home in Pennsylvania for the holidays, when Illa's Christmas card arrived. My mother, who happened to be the postmaster, delivered the card herself and was pleased that I had met someone.

I said we worked with the youth group at our church. No matter how hard I tried to explain that we were just friends, Illa's card caused a lot of excitement among my family and friends.

I flew out of Pittsburgh after the school break and when I deplaned in Chicago, Illa was waiting for me. The surprise turned the frown on my face to a grateful smile. On the way home we talked about the card and me having a new girlfriend from Wheaton. Illa was amused by all the commotion it caused.

Our friendship grew to become something special. Yet, any relationship had limitations because of my bladder condition. As hard as I tried, I always worried about the urine smell. Illa didn't seem to mind and started to wait for me at church if I needed to change clothes. Gradually, we waited for each other.

It became increasingly clear that Illa was interested in me, at least more interested than her parents. Mr. Lebo liked me well enough as a counselor, but Illa's mother was always a little uneasy around me. I knew from past experiences that some parents didn't want their daughters to go out with me because of my physical disability. Many times I'd come very close to asking her for a date, but was afraid to lose the great relationship we had.

Dean Johnson was our youth pastor and had played baseball at Wheaton College with my brother Tommy. Once when he came over to the college to visit me, I asked him about Illa and told him how I felt. Our friendship was special and he was easy to talk to, so I asked him, "Do you think Illa's parents would object to me dating their daughter?"

"I'm pleased that you are interested in her. She is one of the nicest girls I know, Jim. I'll ask her parents if it is all right for you to date her."

It took me a long time to build up my courage to ask her for a date. I had faced rejection all too often. Finally, one Sunday after the youth meeting, we were standing in the hall by ourselves. "Wait a minute, Illa. I want to ask you something."

"Yes, what's on your mind?" She waited a long time for me to ask my question. My mind was embroiled with memories of ridicule and rejection.

Finally, I asked, "Would you go out with me for a milk shake after church?"

To my surprise she said, "Yes, I would like that." I stood there for a long time not knowing what to do.

"What's the matter?"

"No one ever said 'yes' before," I said. "You're the first one who did. I didn't know what to do next. Usually the answer is no and I just walk away." She just laughed.

After church we went to The Seven Dwarfs, a popular college hangout. Over milk shakes I asked her if she wanted to go to the basketball game on Friday. "I have to work the game, but as soon as my work is done I can come and sit with you." She agreed to go and gave me directions to her home.

By Friday I had lost her directions and, relying on my memory, turned down the wrong road. I drove around for a long time, wondering what she would think of me. Since I was an hour and a half late, Illa and her Uncle Bill formed a search party. They were as unsuccessful at finding me as I was at finding the house and by chance, we pulled into her driveway about the same time.

I had allowed extra time before the game, but since I was so late, there was just enough time for brief introductions to Illa's relatives before we had to leave.

At the gym Illa sat in the bleachers and I reported to the equipment room. When the basketball team had everything they needed, I joined Illa until the half. For the second half, Illa and I watched Wheaton continue their winning streak. After the game one the players said his girlfriend was visiting for the weekend and had a friend with her and asked me if I wanted a date. To his surprise, I already had one.

35

During my first six months as equipment manager, I faced a barrage of criticism. I had been doing the job, as I understood it, to the best of my ability and my frustration was mounting. I heard repeatedly how I was not doing the job the way he wanted it done, but was given no direction on how to do it. Finally I said, "I want to please you, but if you're not satisfied, maybe you should find someone else."

As usual he just walked away without a word. Maybe he kept me on because of my devotion to the players. He saw at the games how hard I worked and even though I was the equipment manager, I went beyond and performed some of the trainer's duties.

One day, when Coach seemed in a better mood, I asked him, "What am I doing wrong? How do you want things done?" He just looked at me and didn't answer. "You say I have to do a better job, but you haven't taken the time to explain how you want it done. I'm doing the best I can and unless I understand what's wrong, it won't get any better than this."

I had told him this many times before, but at least this time he didn't yell at me, he just turned and walked away.

About a week later, he called me into his office and showed me a side of himself I wouldn't have believed existed. I was sure I was in trouble, but to my surprise he handed me a picture of my brother Tommy.

"When you came to this school, people introduced you as Tommy's brother. When Tommy comes back to visit, I want people to introduce him as your brother.

"I want you to do something for me. Many students will be discouraged during their first year here and need someone to talk to. You're a good listener and can help them adjust to their new surroundings."

I agreed to do this and he continued in the same gentle voice, explaining how he wanted each job done. Once I understood what he wanted, I completed the job that way. His attitude change and his kindness made him much easier to work for and gave me the desire to please him more. To me he was worth the effort and I worked hard to show him. Over time we became the best of friends.

At Wheaton College, each class started with a prayer and in the fall of 1960, I had a special prayer. I grew up near Pittsburgh and the Pirates were playing the Yankees in the World Series.

During the game I was working in the gym and would run into the storage room off the gym floor to check the score on TV between tasks.

While the Yankees won their games by large margins, the Pirates would eke out a victory by only one or two runs. Pittsburgh didn't rely on a couple of star players to win games. In a close game, many of their players could come through at just the right time.

In the seventh game of the series, the score was tied when the Pirates took the field in the bottom of the ninth. I watched

Bill Mazeroski stroll to the plate, mesmerized by the moment. What happened next broke my trance. "Yahoo! The Pirates win."

As soon as I yelled, the P.E. class in the gym knew what had happened. The students knew where I was from and I was constantly teased about how the Yankees were going to beat the Pirates. "How can you be a Pirate fan?" they asked. "Nothing good ever came from Pittsburgh."

"Lots of good things come from Pittsburgh. I'm here and I'm good," I answered, with humility.

When Jack Schwartz, the P.E. teacher entered the storage room, I said, "Mazeroski hit a home run to win the game and the World Series."

"Well, that was good timing. I had just said, 'Amen' to the prayer, when I heard you yelling." Coach Schwartz was so pleased with my response to the Pirates' victory that he went in and told my boss, Coach Chrouser. Coach was also pleased and had a sign made up for me to put in front of the cage. The sign said, "Jimmy's Pirates win the World Series."

Coach Chrouser gave me a box of Hershey candy bars to hand out to the athletes at the afternoon practice. They thought I provided the candy and thanked me. "Don't thank me," I said, "these are from Coach Chrouser. He wanted the Pirates to win. You know how he hates the Yankees." Still the players found it hard to believe that the coach would do something nice for them.

Coach Chrouser would do everything he could to make the athletes think I was responsible for all the nice things that happened in the gym. He wanted them to think I was someone special and they could talk to me about their problems.

We had reached the point where the coach's comments were about the job I was doing and not about me personally. He had high standards and expected them to be met. He wanted things done right the first time with no time wasted doing things that weren't needed. He made me a great equipment manager and with his training, I believe I could have gone to a professional team.

36

The annual Wheaton College football banquet and awards ceremony was held at the end of the season. This special event called for a special date so I asked Illa to go with me and she accepted.

Coach Chrouser called me into his office. Seeing all of the other coaches there, I was confused and curious. Coach Chrouser smiled broadly. "Jimmy, we have a problem here. Someone ordered this beautiful orchid. The man from the flower shop was told to deliver it to the Centennial gym, but he didn't say who to give it to. Do you have any ideas?"

I knew I had ordered one for Illa, but I wasn't going to tell Coach. Keeping a close eye on me, he took the card from the flower and fumbled with it a little. The other coaches smiled as they watched me squirm. The more I sweated, the more they enjoyed themselves. "How many dates have you had with this lady?" Coach asked.

"This will be our second date."

"You mean you always buy a girl a beautiful flower like this on the second date?" Flushed with embarrassment I wanted to leave, but with so many people present, it was difficult to escape with my flower. Coach Chrouser was happy for me and when I tried to hide my actions, it really tickled him.

We had a great time at the banquet and afterwards joined the football players at a coffeehouse called the Fickle Pickle. It was the first time Illa and I had been to such a place and we were surprised by how well-dressed and normal-looking the beatniks were. When the guy next to me jumped up and started to recite a poem, I jumped up ready to belt him. I thought he wanted to get Illa's attention. As it turned out I captured the attention of the entire room. Even though I stood facing the poet with my fists up ready for a fight, he seemed to be the only person in the room who didn't notice me. He just recited his poem without interruption.

After our coffee, we all went to the band room in the back of the coffeehouse. My friends were all five feet eight or taller and had to bend and crouch to get around in the room's five-foot ceilings. I could move easily and kept yelling at them. "Come on guys, stand up straight." When we sat down and the music started, it was so loud that I wondered if my hearing would ever clear up. This was a new experience for Illa and me and we had a great time that we'll never forget.

We didn't leave the Fickle Pickle until very late. It was about two in the morning when I finally took Illa home. Her parents were really upset with me as they had every right to be. I felt sorry about this and it was the last time I brought her home so late.

My interest in Illa intensified, becoming more and more serious. She was a very pretty girl with a loving spirit that came from her heart, a beautiful reflection of her parents and her upbringing. Never had I met anyone as special as Illa.

While Illa was going to secretarial school in Rock Island, Illinois, she received a disturbing letter from her mother. Her parents saw how quickly things were happening between us and from the beginning had tried to caution her. They had always hoped Illa would marry someone with a degree in Christian Education and my lack of a degree did not fit their vision of her future.

In the letter Illa was reminded how very unhappy her parents were with our relationship. Her mother explained how mundane Illa's life would be with me and how I couldn't offer her the life she deserved. My bladder control problems were an even greater concern. This would make life difficult and cause Illa a lot of heartache if she married me. From that point on, the letter only got worse. Her mother thought the only reason Illa wanted me was because she couldn't find another guy. The letter really made her angry and she thought I should know how her parents felt.

During Illa's time at school in Rock Island, she would go home for weekends where there was no escape from her parents' complaints about me. After listening to their objections repeatedly, during subsequent weekend visits home, she decided to send me a letter.

I was working in Wisconsin at Honey Rock Camp as the Crafts Teacher when I received the devastating news. It was difficult being 450 miles away from Illa and not being able to discuss it with her. All I could do was sit on my bed and think about what should be done.

In her letter Illa suggested flying to Honey Rock Camp to discuss our relationship and her parents' opposition. When the camp nurse heard about this, she offered to share her cabin during Illa's visit.

I thought about how special it was for someone to care enough about me to make this long trip. I looked forward to seeing Illa and spending time together.

Her parents' feelings were a surprise to me because they had always treated me well and had often invited me to Sunday dinner. We would play Ping-Pong after the meal and have a great time. While they never showed any disrespect toward me, their respect had certain limitations.

I understood their feelings. Still I couldn't forget the worthless feeling in my heart. My life had been a series of rejections because of my physical disability. This might have been a normal response to someone in my situation, but I was growing increasingly intolerant of facing this struggle at every stage of my life.

My very special friend Jim Rudolph came into my cabin ready for supper and saw how angry I was. After supper Jim and I talked about how I should deal with this rejection. Jim asked questions that helped me express my feelings and ease my bitterness. Once my feelings were out in the open, it was much easier to confront the problem.

Jim suggested I show no anger when I see her parents at the end of camp. "They know Illa will share the content of the letter with you. Your first response will be anger and they'll expect you to take it out on them. Continue to treat them with respect. It will make them wonder." That was exactly what I did and I've always appreciated how gentle he was in helping me decide what to do.

Illa came in on Friday night and left the following Sunday. For the entire weekend we shared our feelings and hopes for our future if there was going to be one. While we were at camp, Illa and I made a lot of plans. We didn't know if any of them would work out, but we had faith that someday they would materialize. We crammed a lot of discussion and fun into those two days. This time spent together reassured us and strengthened our commitment.

When Illa returned home she tried to change her parents' mind, but no matter what she said, her parents' feelings never changed. My bladder problem was an embarrassment to them, as well as my physical disability. Illa's mother was determined that I would never marry her daughter.

Illa was the most important person in my life, and by this point, we had decided we wanted to be together forever. Moving slowly, we prayed we would find a solution with God directing our thoughts. We hoped God would find a way to make her parents happy with our decision, but it never happened.

We were fighting tremendous odds and her parents' hard feelings only increased the pressure. This drove us even closer together, making us more considerate of each other. We were determined to make each other happy no matter how bad the situation became.

37

Wheaton and North Central Colleges were ten miles apart and bitter rivals. I was at the Centennial gym packing my equipment for the football game against North Central, when one of our track stars came to the equipment room to exchange his dirty clothes for clean ones. I handed him a bundle of laundered clothes: t-shirt, shorts, socks, and jock.

Thadde threw them back at me and yelled, "I don't want these. Give me new clothes."

No one else had problems with the clean clothes I gave them, but Thadde thought he was a star and deserved better treatment. This was the wrong attitude to take and I was determined to treat him like everyone else.

"You'll take what I give you."

"If you don't give me new clothes, I'll have your job."

"Thadde, you wouldn't know how to do this job if you had it. You're not going to get any new stuff."

He went to the coaches' room and brought the coach back to the cage where I worked. "What's going on here, Jimmy?" the coach asked.

I told him what Thadde wanted and said, "Coach, look at what I gave him. Do you see anything wrong with it?"

He looked at the equipment and said, "Just give him a new bundle."

The coach turned to walk away and I was left to stare at Thadde's sarcastic grin. Finding this situation intolerable I said, "Coach, the clothes I gave him are good enough. If you want him to have a new bundle, you can give it to him yourself."

Coach glared at both of us. "Look, I don't have time for this childish nonsense. In case you've forgotten, there is a game this afternoon. Thadde, just take what he gave you. Beating North Central is more important than your jock strap."

He stormed off and yelled, "Jimmy, we're out of towels, bring some back to the coaches' room."

I gathered the towels and Thadde walked back to his locker at the end of the aisle. As I walked by him to the coach's locker room, with my arms full of towels, Thadde jumped me from behind and the towels flew all over the floor.

The football players were getting ready for their game and when they saw this, they surrounded us waiting to intervene. Thadde was taller and heavier, but I was too fast for him and turned around before he had a good hold on me.

I grabbed him under his arms, lifted him off the ground and pinned him against the wall.

"Put me down or I'll kick you between the legs where it hurts."

"If you kick me, I'll bounce your head off the cement, so hard that when you look straight ahead, you'll be looking through your chest."

The football players realized the crisis had passed and returned to their lockers. Thadde had underestimated my strength and wasn't sure what to do next. Finally when his anger subsided, I released him, picked up the towels and carried them to the coach's room.

"Jimmy, what was the disturbance in the locker room?"

"Don't worry about it, Coach, I took care of it." I left and went back to the cage to continue my checklist for the upcoming game.

Thadde had dressed quickly and left the locker room by the time the coach and his assistants came out and asked the players what had happened. "Thadde jumped Jimmy from behind because he didn't get what he wanted. Jimmy moved fast and pinned him against the wall."

Another player added, "We stood by to protect Jimmy and when we saw Thadde pinned against the wall, we knew it was over."

Coach walked out with the players and asked more questions about the incident. He wanted to be sure I wasn't hurt. The players told him, Thadde was very lucky he didn't get the beating of his life. They said I may not be very big, but all of them were smart enough not to mess with my huge arms. One of the players wondered if Thadde learned anything that day, but no one was sure.

Thadde was called into the coach's office on Monday. When he arrived the coach closed the door and asked about the fight. Coach told him if he didn't apologize to me he'd be off the track team. He was given until the following Friday to think about it.

A couple of days later Thadde came into the locker room to see me. "Jimmy, may I talk to you?"

I was working in the cage and answered, "Sure, come on in."

He walked into the cage and said, "Jimmy, I've come to apologize to you for the way I acted on Saturday. Will you accept my apology?"

"Sure Thadde. Thanks."

"You know, I thought for sure you were going to throw me through the wall. I couldn't believe how hard I hit it. I thought I would leave an imprint."

"I'm sorry I hit you so hard. I just lost my temper. If you had asked me nicely, I would have been more likely to give you what you wanted. Instead you came in demanding things with that smirk on your face. So I was determined to treat you like everyone else. Fairly, but like everyone else."

After that Thadde and I became friends and he always kidded me about being so small. He would see me outside and yell, "Hey Jimmy, why don't you get out of that hole in the ground?"

"I like it down here."

"What are you going to be when you grow up?"

"Probably a track star like you."

The football players continued to tease me about how, if I didn't treat them right, I'd have to deal with Thadde.

Sometimes Thadde would hear this, but he took it good-naturedly and soon the jokes moved on to fresher topics.

38

Wheaton had a great football team in 1960 in part because of our short, huge fullback known as Bull. When he ran through the line, he'd knock down anyone in his way. As soon as Bull got the ball, three or four players would try to stop him. Bull was fast and ran so close to the ground, he was difficult to tackle.

In a game with North Central, on the first series of downs, Bull ran the ball and was tackled so hard, every ligament was pulled from one of his knees, requiring surgery. The school doctor told the football coach a couple weeks later, "If someone massages Bull's legs, you could have him for the rest of the season." Coach Chrouser came in and asked me to give Bull the massage.

I had never done anything like this before so the coach explained the procedure. First, I put Bull's legs in the whirlpool to stimulate his circulation. Then I massaged them and put on hot packs to increase the circulation even more. Following a rest, I massaged his legs again before they went back to the whirlpool and I repeated the steps. Each session in the morning and afternoon took about two hours.

Using the whirlpool and hot packs helped to relax and desensitize the muscles. The warmth brought the blood supply to the surface of the skin making the massage easier. The coach always said, "Don't apply too much pressure." When I did, I could feel Bull's muscles contract. The pressure must be firm but gentle. The friction plus the warm oil helped to increase the circulation, which is why the massage works so well.

When Coach Chrouser allowed me to work on the injured athlete, he didn't realize what a tremendous gift he had given me. This opportunity changed my life.

Spina bifida had robbed the strength from my back and legs, so God replaced it with His healing touch working through me.

The pain radiating into my fingertips guides my pressure so I do not inflict pain. With my sensitive touch, I'm able to follow a muscle spasm like a road map.

I was pleased to be useful and able to show God's love. Whenever anyone felt relief from my treatment, God deserved the credit for their healing. I didn't know how to heal anyone. God did it all; I was only His instrument.

I worked on Bull for about three weeks, until his knee was strong enough and he could return to practice. His dedication was the reason the team was so successful. He became stronger and more determined with each game he played. His spiritual strength was an inspiration to all of us, though not the exception. It was typical of the athletes of Wheaton College. Bull and I had a tremendous relationship and God had blessed us both.

Bull was so impressed with how quickly the Lord had healed him that he told everyone, "If you have a problem, go and see Jimmy Byron. He will take care of you and it won't hurt." His faith in me brought other athletes to see me about their injuries. They made me feel they couldn't get along without me.

At the end of the football season, the team held their annual banquet and the players chose Bull for the most valuable player award. Coach Chrouser called him to the front of the room and presented the plaque. Bull thanked those who voted for him and added, "This award should go to Jimmy Byron. He worked so hard to get me ready to play and if he hadn't I would have finished the season on the bench and someone else would be standing here now. We are all fortunate to have someone like Jimmy."

I was surprised and honored that he would give me so much credit. He really deserved the award and set an example for all of us, not allowing his unfortunate injury to stop him. The team was blessed to witness his beautiful attitude and spiritual toughness.

Other injured athletes saw what God had done for Bull and came to me for help. When my regular work responsibilities were completed, I worked on the players. This was the beginning of my ministry with injured athletes. Seeing the relief the athletes derived from my treatments, I became convinced God had shown me what He wanted me to do with my future.

39

When Wheaton College and North Central met again, during the next season in 1961, both teams were ready and couldn't wait to wage war. At that time the teams were on the same sideline with only twenty yards separating each team's bench. When a North Central player came off the field, staggering all over the sideline, I tried to take him by the arm to lead him to his bench. He looked dazed and disoriented as he pulled away from me and swung. He missed me and I tried again to guide him to his bench. Though our actions and reactions occurred repeatedly, his team and coaches did not see that he was hurt.

Finally, he swung and fell to the ground. North Central called a timeout and one of their coaches approached our bench. I ran over to our bench, placed some ice in a towel, dipped the towel in cold water, ran over and applied it to the huge cut he had near his eye. He relaxed and there was no further resistance.

The Wheaton College Chaplain knelt beside him and prayed until the ambulance came and the player was taken up to the Wheaton Infirmary. After the game three of our players went to see how their injured opponent was doing.

As soon as they introduced themselves he asked, "Did you see that midget on the field?"

"No, we didn't see a midget on the field."

"The really short guy?"

"Oh, you mean Jimmy."

"You know, I took a swing at him."

"That's okay, Jimmy, won't think anything about it."

"I didn't mean to do that."

"I'm sure he's forgiven you. Anyway, we just came in to see how you're doing." After a short visit, they left allowing the injured athlete to rest.

The next day, after church, they went back to see him again. He was told that it was important for him to meet their special friend. "I don't see anyone but you guys."

"Well, He's with us, but you can't see Him."

"If he's with you, how come I can't see him?"

"His name is Jesus Christ and He is very interested in you. He loves you and will be with you in all that you do. We want you to accept Jesus Christ as your savior."

They spent the afternoon telling him how Jesus had made their lives better. After leaving the infirmary, they stopped by my room to tell me about the guy who had swung at me. I was at Illa's house that Sunday and didn't learn about it until Monday.

The players believed my placing the ice pack on our injured opponent's face was the act of kindness that made him so receptive to their words. They were really excited and gave me most of the credit.

I told them I would do this for anyone in need of help. Someone thought my act of compassion and the chaplain praying over the player was so special that they took a picture of all three of us.

I've always treasured that picture because it dramatizes the core of my Christian faith. Later, when our family moved to Springfield, I found the picture and thought it could represent the central theme of my massage business. I would develop my spiritual touch as a masseur, on the love that Christ gives to all of us.

I had this picture enlarged to a wall-size poster with the inscription, "Healing Power Comes from Love, Love Comes from Christ." I made a commitment to God to reach out and touch the hearts of others. I have never taken credit for God's healing and He has blessed my service as a masseur now for over fifty years.

40

Illa finished secretarial school and her parents decided she should study to become a nurse. This was their latest effort to keep us apart and was a tough time for Illa. She felt the teachers went through the material too fast and it was difficult for her to understand what was being said. With constant pressure to get good grades and unfavorable comparisons to her successful older brother, Illa grew to hate school. When she decided she didn't want to be a nurse, her parents' angry response demoralized her.

Illa called to tell me she wasn't going back to school and we agreed to meet at the Wheaton College homecoming. While my family waited at the restaurant I told Mom, Illa was really down and her parents were angry with her for quitting nursing. Illa was still upset when she came into the restaurant and Mom could see the disappointment in her eyes. "Illa, come sit by me," Mom said and treated her with so much love that she felt special.

We went bowling and had a great time with my family. Illa said she could see why I loved my mother so much. Even though she was not part of the family, she felt more at home than she did with her own family.

After she quit school, we both felt it was a good time to make plans for our wedding. Illa's friend, Mr. White was the manager of the campus book store where Illa worked. The store also carried jewelry and he helped us pick out an engagement ring and our wedding rings.

Before I could expect Illa to become my wife, I had to know how she felt about my lack of bladder control. I picked her up after work and on the way home I gave her the engagement ring. We discussed bladder control issues and despite these problems, she accepted the ring and agreed to marry me. It was the happiest day of my life.

Illa told her parents about our decision to get married. We saw this as the beginning of a great life, but knew we would have a very difficult time with her parents. They responded with anger and redoubled their efforts to end our relationship. From this point on, our problems escalated. When Illa told her parents she was going to see my mother to discuss our upcoming marriage, they forbade her to go.

We went to Pennsylvania, without her parents' permission or blessing. My mother had invited us to come home to discuss our plans. My brother Shun lived in Wheaton and I often talked to him about marrying Illa. He had shared what I had told him with Mom, which made our meeting easier.

My mother was concerned about whether or not we could have children and the problems childlessness could cause. If we wanted children and couldn't have them, it could ruin our marriage. She advised us to see a doctor about this.

After seeing a doctor, we learned there was nothing wrong and we should be able to have children. In fact, the doctor who was a good friend of mine thought we would have a pretty normal marriage and encouraged us. When we called my mother to share the news, she told us this was her main concern. She was happy for both of us and gave us her blessing.

After Illa's parents realized our marriage was inevitable, they grudgingly accepted the situation. With her mother's help, they went to look at apartments. Some of them were terrible, but they found one that had just been completed and the rent was within our budget. Next they looked for furniture and cleaned the apartment before we moved in. They both worked very hard to make the place look nice.

With my future mother-in-law's strong negative feelings about me, I was stunned when she was so helpful. I knew this had nothing to do with me. Her only desire was to make her daughter happy. They even bought her a new wardrobe for the wedding.

Illa's mother planned the wedding, decorated the church basement, and made the punch for the reception. Everything was done with such care and looked great. The Lebos worked hard to make everything successful. They provided a delicious rehearsal dinner at their home. Hope Lebo was one of the best cooks I've ever known. There was plenty of food, even enough for my brothers' tremendous appetites.

I moved into the apartment two weeks before we were married. During the weekend of the wedding, my mother and brothers stayed with me at the apartment. We had a great time together and they couldn't understand why I wasn't feeling nervous. What they didn't realize was that I was scared to death.

There was also time for private talks with Mom. She wanted to know a little more about Illa, which gave me the opportunity to talk about my favorite subject. "Illa is probably the most beautiful girl I've ever met. As pretty as she is, her real beauty comes from her heart. I love her very much and we want to be together always. As long as we're together, we can handle any problems we face."

"Your dad and I were the same way. I wish he could be here for the wedding. I'm very proud of you and Dad would be too."

"I often wonder why Dad is gone and I'm still here. As I look back, I'm the one with the physical disability and Dad could have accomplished so much more if he could have lived longer."

"I don't know why God took Dad home. In many ways he lives on through us and we all must do our best to make our lives count."

I wasn't expected to live long and not much had ever been asked of me. No one wanted me to succeed more than my mother did. Now I felt, in both my marriage and my life, I had a duty to fulfill. My tears were so heavy it was difficult to see Mom.

After she left, I stayed in my room until the tears dried. All I could think of was having Dad at the wedding. We had chosen Mom and Dad's favorite hymn, "In the Garden" for our ceremony. This way, even though Dad wasn't there, he would not be forgotten.

On our wedding day, I was surprised to see such a crowded church. Illa and I were very fortunate to have so many friends.

When Illa came down the aisle, I could not take my eyes off her. She was so radiant, the most beautiful sight I'd ever seen, and this angel was mine. The Lord really blessed me with a very special girl and I knew I made the right choice.

We spent the first night at a motel in Aurora, Illinois and the next morning went on to Rochester, Minnesota. My Brother Jack's wife, Lois was sick and unable to attend the wedding, so Illa and I decided to pay them a surprise visit.

In Jack's neighborhood, we saw some young kids playing and asked them where Jack Byron lived.

"I'll show you," one said.

"How do you know him?" I asked.

"He's my dad," the boy smiled, "I'll show you where our house is Uncle Jim."

I hadn't seen my nephew, Jamie since he was a toddler and didn't recognize him. When we entered the house, we saw Jack and Lois with my mother and Aunt Louise. Everyone was surprised to see us. Since Lois had missed our wedding, she was especially delighted that we had made the trip. For two days Illa got to know my family better and everyone seemed pleased with our marriage.

We spent the remainder of our honeymoon back at our new apartment, which at this point was not yet fully furnished. Soon we found a dirty old white refrigerator. We wanted to make it look better so we asked our landlord for permission to paint it inside the apartment.

He said he didn't care, so we moved the refrigerator to the middle of the room to make the job easier. With a can of bright yellow spray paint, we sprayed it once and waited for it to dry. The first coat did little to cover the dirt. For the second coat, we grew careless and when we were finished we had not only painted the refrigerator but also the chairs, sink, table and everything else in the kitchen.

Before we started, the apartment looked so nice and with just two coats of paint, we changed all that. When we showed the landlord what we had done, I offered to repaint the kitchen. With an amused grin he declined my offer and said he'd take care of it. He teased us for months following this incident, offering to bring in more refrigerators for us to paint.

Mr. Shimp was the nicest landlord. Seeing him on the front stoop, we would stop to visit. We struggled with his name, calling him Simp, or Shrimp. He seemed as amused with his new names as we were in messing up his real one.

41

With the exception of a similarity of their names, Dr. Barabus had little in common with the thief Barabbas from the Passion story. He was a professor of Bible Studies at Wheaton College and an avid tennis player. His interest in the sport resulted in a sprained ankle which left him hobbling between classes on crutches.

A football player saw this and told him I might be able to help. My massages in the training room were becoming known throughout the school. When the professor came over to discuss this with me, I told him at this point I had only worked on athletes and would check with the coach.

With the coach's permission, I began the professor's massages in the Centennial gym the following Monday. His ankle and foot were very tender, so I massaged only his legs for the first few days. This was done three for four times each day before placing his feet in the whirlpool. This helped to relieve a lot of tension. Results came slowly, but by the end of the first week, his need for crutches diminished and by Monday, he was only using a cane.

We continued for another week and when he came in to see me the following Monday, he was excited by his progress. He could not believe how much he had improved by the end of the second week and was even able to play tennis.

"Jim, The Lord has blessed you with a beautiful gift. Don't waste it. What you need now is the training to go with your touch."

He wrote to a number of schools and finally chose a school of Swedish massage in downtown Chicago. Illa and I went to the school to observe a class. My major concern was my ability to comprehend the written material and retain the information. Mrs. Swanson was an elderly Swedish woman and we hit it off right away. She had been teaching massage for twenty-seven years and knew all about it, so I decided to take the course. At home Illa and I spent a great deal of time going over the different techniques, endlessly practicing.

Mrs. Swanson took an interest in me and I received a lot of individual instruction. Every time I gave a massage, she was looking over my shoulder, though her corrections were never unkind. Whenever I made a mistake, she pointed it out and showed me how correct it. I took advantage of this by asking questions until I understood the right technique.

After completing the ten-month course, there was a written test and a performance portion where the student gave the instructor a massage. This was her way of knowing if you understood what you were doing and had mastered the techniques. If you failed the test, you did not receive a diploma.

When I finished the massage, she told me it was the best one she had had in twenty-seven years. She was a large woman and I was able to give her a good massage because I was used to working on my massaging partner who was built like a linebacker. My ability had increased each week because of the energy and strength I developed giving him massages.

"You have tremendous strength in your hands and fingers," the instructor said and added how rare it was for an individual to have a touch as strong as mine and still be gentle enough not to hurt anyone. "Be careful not to apply too much pressure. You have a great future ahead of you. Use it wisely."

I knew my gift had come from God and I decided to do whatever He wanted me to do with it. God had finally found a niche for me. This was the beginning of a ministry that would last for years, giving tremendous purpose to my life. Thanks to Dr. Barabus's belief in me and hope for my future, I was directed to the massage school where I gained the knowledge to pursue God's work.

During my massage class I learned when a muscle is dormant for a long time, it will not develop. While the instructor talked about this, I thought about my bladder control problem and decided to try to develop my muscles to achieve continence. I tired quickly wearing the urinal and to go through life without it would be such a blessing. Incontinence was just another situation I'd have to work through.

The next day I discussed this with Coach Chrouser in the equipment room. I explained what I wanted to do and the ill effects we were likely to encounter. Training my muscles to control my bladder would be a difficult challenge. Since I planned to stop wearing my urinal, smelly accidents were sure to occur. Reaching my goal could take a very long time and I needed everyone's patience and support. The coach suggested I address the players at their weekly prayer meeting that evening.

At the prayer meeting I was nervous about asking for their understanding and patience. I knew the smell of urine was repulsive and I was embarrassed to discuss my plan with the athletes. They had no problem with bladder control themselves, but after I explained my struggles with this problem, they appreciated the challenges I faced. When I finished, the players told me how they admired the courage it took for me to speak to them. At the end of the meeting, we formed a circle and their prayers lifted my spirit.

At subsequent meetings, the athletes continued to pray for me and I always thanked them and said what a difference their prayers made. This generosity increased my desire to continue and not give up.

I practiced by tightening my stomach muscles and holding this position as long as I could. This would eventually improve my control, but the process sent spasms to my muscles. Each day my bladder control improved, but on bad days, lines of exhaustion marked my face as I strained to control myself. Many times I'd have to wash and rinse my clothes to minimize the smell. God always sent someone to encourage me and I always felt tomorrow would be better. After about eight months, I felt energized and happy to be free of the urinal.

During an insurance physical, my doctor asked why I wasn't wearing my urinal. I told him about my experiment and everyone's support and prayers. He was pleased with my accomplishment and told me if I had asked him about this, he would have told me what I had done was impossible. All I could say was: "Then I'm sure glad that I didn't ask you."

Coach Chrouser often asked how I was getting along during this period and when I achieved my goal, told me how proud he was of me. I have always believed the athletes' kindness and compassion were a reflection of Coach Chrouser's leadership. When I asked him once if he spoke to the captains of the football team about my problem, he just smiled and walked away.

42

After a year of marriage and the desire to have children someday, we decided we needed to find a larger apartment as nice as the one we had. Illa's parents decided we should buy a house. We were having a difficult time paying our rent and I didn't know how we would be able to afford the mortgage payments. As usual, my opinion meant nothing. They were determined to buy a house for their daughter and any future grandchildren. While we would make the payments, they would choose the house and make the down payment.

The four of us went to talk to a realtor. This gave her father the opportunity to publicly embarrass me. He made it clear to the realtor that they were buying this house for their daughter and I would have no say in the transaction.

Over a two-month period, we looked at a few houses until finally Illa's mother found a house she liked in West Chicago and as usual, her husband agreed with her. Illa and I liked the house too, but of course, my opinion didn't matter.

After they bought the house, Illa's father told me I could do nothing to the house without their permission, not even repairs. So, with the exception of mowing the grass, I did nothing around the house.

My father-in-law quickly tired of making repairs and told me I could have fixed some of the small problems. When I reminded him I was not allowed to do anything, he got angry and told me I was worthless. No matter what I did, it was never good enough. We often exchanged sharp words and our tempers were ready to explode at any time.

Illa's brother and sister-in-law, George and Kathy were visiting from Florida and we were invited to Illa's parents' house to see them. I had a church softball game, so on the way I dropped Illa off and planned to join them later.

When I returned home after the game to shower, I was surprised to find Illa home and crying. Her visit started out fine, but soon escalated into a fight. Compliments about the cleanliness of her mother's house led to sarcastic comments about Illa's housekeeping abilities. Illa's mother was relentless and finally Illa had enough. She stormed out of the house and headed down the road for home.

It soon became clear that Illa was not coming back. Her father was sent to retrieve her and when he found her, he told her to get in the car. Illa refused and her father grabbed her, trying to make her come back. She agreed to get in the car when her father promised to take her home.

Illa's explanation of these events was interrupted by the phone. I answered it and Illa's mother asked if we were coming back to see George and Kathy. I couldn't believe she would ask this. She acted as though nothing had happened.

"No, we're not coming over because of the way you treated Illa. George and Kathy can come over here if they want to see us."

"I was simply pointing out how she might improve. I always treat my daughter with love. Illa just exaggerates things."

"No, Illa doesn't. She told me what you said. We will not be over." My voice rose in a crescendo of aggravation until I slammed the phone down and Illa resumed her account.

My anger probably confirmed Illa's parents' belief that she had married the wrong person. I knew my relationship with my in-laws would not improve until they started treating her with kindness and respect. Illa was my wife and I didn't want anyone to hurt her in any way. I was taught no matter how tough a problem is I had to work on it. Throughout my life I had to learn how to overcome obstacles and make adjustments.

Later her mother called again. By this time tempers had cooled and Illa agreed to go back and we enjoyed our time with George and Kathy.

Our house did not have a garage and one day after work Illa informed me that a man was coming over to talk about building one next to the house. "We can't afford it," I said.

"Well, he's coming over. Mom and Dad invited him."

"That's nice. Since the house belongs to your parents, do I have to be here?"

"I'd like you to be here and see what he has to say."

When her parents came over I said, "It would have been nice if we had discussed this first."

"We are doing this for our daughter and you have no say in the matter."

I had heard this so many times in the past and was sick of hearing it. Shaking my head in desperation, I turned and walked away.

The man came in and showed us pictures of the garage, explaining all the features. I was quiet during this time and only spoke when he asked me a question. It bothered me that I was expected to be grateful for this intrusion in our financial affairs. My in-laws never cared about how I felt. If my feelings were hurt, they were sure I'd soon get over it.

When the salesman finished his presentation, he asked me if I had any questions.

"No, my wife's parents are putting up the garage. I have no say in what they do. They're paying for it."

When the man left, I could see Illa's parents were angry. Her mother said, "Try to contain your gratitude."

"I want to provide for my wife without outside interference."

"Well, we'll interfere no longer," she said. "Come on, George, we're leaving."

For the first time that day I was grateful.

We often heard how Illa made the wrong choice when she married me. Being viewed as a mistake didn't help my attitude.

As much as I hated to miss church, there were times when the pain in my back was so severe that I couldn't get out of bed. Whenever I had to miss church, Illa's parents called to ask where I was. I had explained this to them many times, but they never seemed to believe me. During our first years of marriage, we couldn't make a move without some sarcastic comments from her parents. Finally I'd had enough and when this happened I'd just walk away.

Illa's mother must have seen this as a sign of weakness and with this taste of blood, her attacks intensified. I was always on the defensive so I had to stand up for myself by responding to every criticism and insult.

This tension could not continue. We had to find a way to work things out and get along together. I had to learn to control my anger and work toward a brighter future. It would take me a long time, but friendlier family relations would be worth the effort.

43

I was working long hours at the college for low wages and had long believed our house was too expensive. Illa and I also wanted to have a child so I felt we needed more income. I had been working at the college for over four years without a pay increase, so I asked Coach for a raise.

"How much do you need?" he asked.

"I would like an extra ten dollars a month."

"I can't afford that much of an increase."

"Well, I need more money. If you can't give it to me, I'll have to go somewhere else."

"You won't be able to find a job better than this."

I was angry with Coach and needed someone to talk to. My brother Tommy worked at the Student Union, so I went over to tell him I was going to look for another job. I asked if he thought I was doing the right thing. Tommy knew we needed more money and was behind me all the way.

After a while, I thought the Coach was right about the difficulty I would have finding a new job. I looked for about six months without success. Finally, I went to a private agency for help. It didn't take long before I had an interview for a cashier position at the Pontiac dealership in Wheaton. The job paid $40.00 more per year than I made working at the college, but the increase was only a third of what I'd asked Coach for. After the interview, I was offered the job and I accepted.

I went back to the college to give Coach my two-week notice. He was really angry and said I couldn't leave.

"You said no one would hire me. You were wrong."

"Didn't you know I was kidding?"

"No, I didn't and the income I need to support my family is a serious manner."

"Will you reconsider?"

"I've already accepted. It's too late now."

"What am I supposed to do on such short notice?"

"I don't know. You should have thought about that when I asked for a raise."

By my last day, his anger had subsided and he threw a little party for me. We parted friends and stayed in touch for many years.

Six months after I left Wheaton College, I resumed work on injured athletes in my home for free. One of the players called and said he was hurt and asked if I could help him. After just a couple of massages, Bob was able to go back to practice. This was much quicker than we had thought and, like in the past, I was convinced God had healed him through my hands. Bob asked if he could continue to see me and bring friends who were also injured.

I talked to Illa and she agreed this was an opportunity to share our love. We prayed for guidance and believed God lead us to pursue this ministry on a regular basis.

We lived ten miles from the school and during the first couple of weeks, I made four or five trips per week to pick up a group of players at the dorm. They enjoyed getting away from the school and we had fun too. God really blessed our time together.

The players knew we were home most evenings and when they got cars, they would often drop by for a visit. Sometimes, we'd have a couple of players over for dinner. After football practice they were starved and we didn't have leftovers on those nights. We were delighted to share what we had with them and they were as pleased as we were.

Not only did the players' cars increase their mobility, I no longer had to pick them up for their massages. Bob would always call first to get my permission and tell me how many were coming. On one visit I noticed a newcomer who was very quiet and seemed troubled. Bob had told me he was an excellent athlete and was well liked by the players. I knew something was disturbing him but I didn't know what it was.

Like with each new person, I explained how the Lord had given me this talent to be used on injured athletes and I offered to work on him.

He just laid there and didn't say anything. It was easy to see he was hurting inside so I told him, "I don't know what's bothering you and it's none of my business. I want you to know that I really love you. The Lord has touched my heart and I want to share my feelings with you. You are very special. Don't forget that."

After the massage we had cake and ice cream and the athletes went back home. When the young man went into the dorm, he told his friends what I had said to him and their discussion ran late into the night. The athletes came back the next day to tell me what had happened. His mother and father had filed for a divorce and called after football practice to tell him. He didn't know it was coming and it was a devastating blow. My kind words were just what he needed to hear and the players believed the Lord had used me to touch this man's heart.

At the end of 1964 season, Bob invited us to the Wheaton College football banquet. Illa and I were pleased to go and it was a great dinner. We enjoyed the fellowship and felt special to be included.

As one of the team's co-captains, Bob gave a speech to honor a very special person who always gave his time to help others. I knew he was talking about Coach Bubba who everyone loved and related to.

"Jimmy, will you come up to the front of the room?" I looked around at all the people to see who he was talking about. I just sat there until Illa nudged me.

I walked up and joined Bob at the podium. He turned to me he said, "We've come out to your home during the football season and you never charge us for your service. We know you won't take any money, but you will be a father soon, so we have this hundred dollar savings bond in your daughter Mary's name. You can't refuse, because you'd be in trouble with Illa."

I was speechless as the audience stood and applauded. When the cheers subsided, I thanked him and returned to my seat. Wow, what a great feeling. God's tremendous love filled the room. I felt humbled by the special blessing of everyone's kindness.

44

When it came time to take Illa to the hospital, I was excited by the thought of becoming a father. My mind was reeling through the checklist of things I needed to do as I backed the car out of the driveway. I stopped suddenly when I heard Illa yell, "Don't you think I should go with you?"

"That sounds like a good idea," I said. Illa got in the car and off we went to the hospital.

From my early childhood, I was not expected to experience the normal joys of life. I was not expected to hold a job, get married, have children, or even live very long.

Hearing Mary's cry from the delivery room filled my heart with endless possibility. Her birth on December 20, 1964 changed everything in our lives.

Everyone had feared that our child would have spina bifida and this became the focus of our prayers. Seeing the nurse approach with Mary, I felt joy and worry all at once. With coal-black hair and soft white skin, she was the most beautiful little girl I'd ever seen. When the nurse told me she was perfectly normal, I could barely contain my excitement and pride.

After church, Illa's folks came to the hospital to see their new granddaughter. I escorted them to the nursery to see Mary and could see the transformation in their eyes. After a while, they returned to Illa's room to visit with her and praise the baby. While Illa rested, they took me out to dinner.

Even though I had missed breakfast, I didn't feel hungry. My father-in-law kidded me about being excited and insisted that I eat something.

"There's no reason to get so excited," he said. "I've seen pigs and cows born many times. This is just another birth. You'll get used to it."

"If you're not excited," I asked, "why are you putting salt in your coffee?" He looked down at his cup very quickly to check and realized I was kidding.

This was a high point in my relationship with my in-laws. All it took was a grandchild to ease the tension between us. Whether my father-in-law admitted it or not, they were excited and loved Mary very much.

After dinner I returned home and called my mother to share the news. "Mary has black hair, soft white skin and is beautiful." Fearing the worst, Mom asked if Mary was all right. "Mom, Mary has no defects at all." I could hear her sigh of relief we both cried with joy.

From the beginning of our very special marriage, I was determined to make Illa happy. I would remind her many times a day how much I loved her and would look for special and unexpected ways to show it. Our feelings were warm and gentle, with a richness that came from Christ. By leading Christian lives, with regular church attendance, we became involved with activities that brought us closer to the Lord and God blessed us with a precious love for each other, which gave our lives an exceptional quality.

THE HEALING TOUCH

The addition of Mary to our family was the answer to our prayers. Her love and sense of humor brought us a new dimension of pleasure and her inner beauty touched our hearts.

Mary was a happy little girl and enjoyed herself in whatever she did. She had so much energy and was into everything. When Mary was old enough to crawl, she would dart from place to place, quickly finding places where she was not supposed to be. By eight months she pulled herself up to the couch, stood for a little while, and started to walk. We thought she was fast when she crawled, but walking even increased her speed.

When I read the Sunday paper, Mary would sneak up, hit the paper, and run away laughing. I'd tell her not to do this, but she kept it up until I chased her around the table.

We were still living in the West Chicago house Illa's parents bought for us, a ranch-style house with an acre of ground. This was Mary's yard to explore and she would run all over and never tire.

We had a huge vegetable garden and Mary always wanted to help. Whenever I put a seed in the ground, my helper would pick it up and hand it back to me. Each time I told her not to do this, she would answer, "Sure Daddy, I can do it," and continued. We both enjoyed the game and had a good time.

When Mary walked into the massage room, the athletes lying on the table couldn't see her. She was very small and would sneak into the room and tickle their feet. Mary loved to see them jump all over the table.

Mary and the athletes had a ball playing together. They passed her toys around and she ran from one person to the next trying to get them. When it was time for them to go, Mary gave them a hug and a kiss and the players looked forward to seeing Mary again.

45

Paying our bills in West Chicago was very difficult. Illa quit her full-time job during her pregnancy and after Mary was born, she returned to work part time in the evenings.

One dark rainy night Illa's boss called and asked if she was coming to work. Her trip up Prince Crossing Road to North Avenue normally took about fifteen minutes and when he learned she had left forty-minutes minutes earlier, we assumed she had had car trouble. I was alone with Mary and without a car so Mike offered to look for Illa.

I called my mother-in-law to see if Illa had stopped there on her way to work. Learning she hadn't, I told her mother what I knew at this point and told her I would call when I knew more.

As soon as I hung up, the phone rang again. A voice told me there had been an accident and when I asked for details he hung up.

I called the hospital and asked if an ambulance brought a woman into emergency? I explained to her that my wife was missing and I was told there had been an accident.

"What is your wife's name?"

"Her name is Illa Byron."

"Yes, she's here."

My brother Shun had a new job in Chicago and was living with us while he looked for an apartment. He arrived home from work about ten minutes later and took me to the hospital where I was immediately taken to the emergency ward to see Illa.

Her broken jaw stuck out from her face, and while I nearly passed out from the sight, she was in good spirits. When I left the emergency room to see my brother, my face was still very white.

I called Illa's mother from the hospital and they came right over. By the time they arrived, the swelling in Illa's face had increased. She looked up at her mother and said, "Hi Mom. I have a swelled head." I could see the pain in their faces as the horrific events of that evening unfolded during our half hour visit. Two cars, neck and neck confronted Illa on the two-lane road, leaving only the soft shoulder as an escape route. Illa had seen the four headlights before she swerved off the road to avoid a head-on collision. The next thing she remembered was giving her phone number to the anonymous stranger. After the paramedics pulled her from the car, she learned the car had rolled over three times flattening the roof before hitting two trees.

The four of us thanked the Lord for Illa's survival and joined in prayer before we left her bedside. Illa's parents took Mary home with them and cared for her until Illa was able to.

I told Shun what I had learned and the next morning I called my mother to tell her about the accident. Mom was very upset and I tried to ease her worries and reassure her that everything would be fine. "Illa's jaw is broken, but her tongue still wags." This eased the tension and Mom laughed.

The doctors told me Illa might have to have surgery to reset her jaw, though there was a possibility the jaw would reset itself. The force of a sneeze could be enough to do this. The need for surgery was averted when Illa expressed a desire for a chocolate milk shake. After Illa's dad brought her one, she became very sick and threw up. Neither of them realized the therapeutic potential of a milk shake, but that was all it took.

Repairing the splintered bone around her left eye was not so simple. That required a long operation. During this time a candy striper kept me company. She was a friend from our church and Illa was her youth leader. We talked about how important Illa was to both of us and we prayed for Illa's recovery. This was a tremendous help to me.

After she left I thought about my life with Illa. We went everywhere together. It would be hard to live without someone so special.

I knew this was a difficult operation because the bone was splintered so badly and the procedure would take a lot out of Illa. So I was relieved when the doctor came in and said she would be all right. This relief was short-lived when he added that a couple of times they almost lost her.

"She doesn't appear to be very strong, but she really fought to stay alive. She must have felt that she had something to live for."

"Yes she does," I said. "It's our family."

As difficult as the operation was and all Illa went through, it further strengthened our marriage. It taught us not to take each other for granted. Illa is still the light of my life and I thank God every day for bringing us together.

46

My mother was on vacation in Raleigh, North Carolina, visiting her oldest son Jack and his wife Lois when she received a call from her brother Mel. After a Wednesday night prayer meeting, his daughter Joann had gone upstairs to check on her five children, turned to go back downstairs, had a heart attack and died. My mother felt Joann's children needed her help more than she needed a vacation, so she decided to go to West Virginia.

Illa's accident had happened less than two months earlier and no one in the family was prepared for the tragedy we were about to face. A policeman called my brother Tug after finding his number in Mom's purse. Tug had already spoken to my brother Jack by the time he reached me at home that evening. About forty miles north of Raleigh, in a severe thunderstorm, Mom lost control of the car. The windshield popped out from the impact of the rolling vehicle and Mom was thrown through the front window before the car landed on top of her.

It was late in the evening before Shun returned home to his Chicago apartment and I broke the news to him. The next day, Illa, Shun, and I left for McGrann. Arriving in our hometown, we met sadness everywhere. She was so much a part of life in this small community. It was difficult for everyone to accept that she was gone forever.

Mom had a great love for young people. She felt there wasn't a bad kid in the world and if you treated them with respect, you would have a friend for life. Young people were our richest blessings and it was our duty to make them feel special.

At the funeral, Reverend Stone shared a story about his brother with the congregation. "My brother was living in Massachusetts when he died and I had no money to go to his funeral. Anne gave me the money for the plane ticket as well as a little spending money while I was there. This was just one way Anne touched my life as she did all of our lives. Anne had a special love for the people in her community. It didn't matter who it was; if she saw someone in need, she would help.

"Anne had a tireless devotion to her family and worked hard to provide for her sons. She had tremendous love for her son Jim."

With my emotions very close to the surface anyway, tears started to come and I couldn't stop them. My uncle, Big Bob, put his arm around my shoulders and I buried my head in his chest. The loss of my mother was devastating. With her love and guidance, I could handle any situation. My mother had the ability to look at difficult problems and find solutions. When I faced personal crises, and there were plenty, I always went to her. She was a great listener, never giving me advice unless I asked for it. She would ask me questions in such a way that it looked like I had made the decision and for many years, I thought I had. Mom was very patient with me and would not only encourage me to stick with my decisions, but helped me to work them out. If I made a mistake, Mom helped me to see what was wrong. Now that she was no longer here, I had to learn to deal with my problems alone.

Mom showed so much love that people felt better just being in her company. She could turn away anger with not only a smile but with great wisdom. Mom was the one who encouraged me in my dream of working with young people.

I've always felt that God had a ministry for me and it was important for me to have the same spiritual impact on young people that my mother had. The Lord gave me the calling and my mother's love lives on through my work.

After the funeral we all shared memories of Mom and our lives together. My brothers explained how concerned Mom was about my spina bifida and the risk of bladder infections. For the first time I realized how central these infections were to my problems.

At times when the pain was so severe, I'd ask my mother what caused it. I sensed how painful my questions were so I stopped asking and just tried to endure in silence. Dr. Winters would tell my brothers that if they didn't measure up to the pain I could handle, that they weren't as tough as I was.

My mother had a very difficult time watching me suffer. She never told me how serious my condition was and never spoke of the possibility of my premature death. Mom taught me to make the most out of life, regardless of what I faced. She told me to live each day as if it were my last and make my life count for something good.

My brothers reminded me of what an important role Dr. Winters had in my life. Whenever he was called, no matter where he was, he would come to see me. The memory of Dr. Winters' thoughtfulness touched my heart and brought tears to my eyes. He made me feel special. When he walked in, he said that he was in the neighborhood and wanted to know how his best patient was doing. He seemed more like a close friend than a doctor, encouraging me not to give up. I knew the reason I was alive was because of his care.

When Illa and I returned home from the funeral, I wrote a letter to Dr. Winters, thanking him for the life he had given me. I stressed how his devotion and love had made the difference. "I want to help others as you have helped me," I wrote. "I will not waste my life. I will make a difference in this world. The Lord will be able to work through me. Whatever comes out of it will be because of your love. I will never forget how very special you are to me. Always remember that I love you."

47

With a growing family the need for more income was an ongoing concern. I worked for a couple of years at the Pontiac dealership, followed by another couple years at Streator Clay Pipe doing clerical work at the Carol Stream office. A move to an assembly line job in a factory in Elmhurst provided another pay increase. After starting the factory job, I heard about an opportunity at the Elmhurst YMCA for a part-time masseur. I was on the day shift, Monday through Friday, so my evenings and weekends were free.

When I went down to apply, I was asked to wait in the lobby. Seated in front of a large picture window, I watched the cars go by and after a few minutes a man sat down and struck up a conversation with me. I shared my interest in sports with him and talked about how important my family was to me and the central role of religion in our lives. After mentioning I was there to apply for a job, I told him I had gone to the Kellberg Institute and had been a volunteer masseur with the athletes at Wheaton College for four years.

At this point I had been talking to this stranger for a long time and I was beginning to wonder when someone would see me about the job. Finally he said, "I like your attitude. My name is Bill and I'm the head of the health club here. I'd like to try you out. Can you start next week?"

"Sure, I can start whenever you want me," I said as he smiled at my surprise. "I didn't even realize I was being interviewed."

"I do my interviews this way because people are generally not aware of what I'm doing. They are relaxed and will give me more honest and candid information. You seem confident and willing to learn, so I'm going to teach you to be a good masseur. If there's something you don't understand I expect you to ask questions. Don't be ashamed to ask. If I don't make sense, keep asking until you understand what I mean."

Bill took me through each procedure step by step until I developed a more relaxed control of my technique. I liked his approach and planned to take full advantage of his instruction. Bill was a perfectionist and when he left me in charge, I was expected to perform at his level.

Bill was very good to me and saw how eager I was to learn. Some of his techniques took time to master and he understood that I was having a difficult time. After years of working on injured athletes, I had developed a soft touch. Bill continued to encourage me to try new techniques to expand my range of treatment for a wider array of problems. He was always patient when I gave him a massage, suggesting changes as I went. After a while Bill finally said, "This is the best massage you've given me yet. I'm really proud of you."

I'll never forget Bill's devotion which inspired me to do my best. He always said, "As good as you are, you want to continue to read about new techniques and try to apply them. Never be satisfied with what you know. You must always strive to improve. If you do this, you'll always be in demand."

Bill was right--I was always in demand. I loved my work and found joy in the people I met. One Saturday, as I was walking into the Health Center, this little boy asked me why I was so small. His mother was very embarrassed, but I told her it was okay. Children are always honest and don't mean anything unkind by their questions. I told him when I was his age, I didn't drink my milk. He walked away from me saying, "I don't want to be short like him."

The next week when I came to work his mother was waiting to thank me. She told me her son wouldn't even touch his milk before he saw me and now he drinks two glasses a day. This story left a smile on my face for the rest of the day.

48

Three years after our daughter Mary was born, we had a baby boy. Bob enjoyed himself and was content in whatever he did. He was very quick and watching him required a good eye. Bob was generally quiet unless he wanted something. Once when he was about a year old, Illa was doing the dishes and he managed to get out of his playpen. The front door was open and Bob took it as an invitation to go out and explore. He went through the door, into the yard and out onto the road. Illa learned of Bob's escape when a driver picked him up and brought him back to the house. This incident really frightened us and from that moment on, we watched Bob more closely.

While visiting Illa's parents when Bob was two, Mary wanted to walk down to the pond to see the ducks. Bob wanted to go too and asked to be carried. Illa told him he was a big boy and if he wanted to go, he had to walk. An angry fit followed and Illa left Bob in the yard under my watchful eye. With Illa, Grandma and Mary gone, Bob's anger grew. He was sitting underneath a couple of hickory trees and made so much noise that the agitated squirrels ran through branches, raining twigs and nuts on top of his head. At this Bob's anger rose to the next level. When his grandfather told him not to hurt the squirrels, Bob didn't think Grandpa was very funny.

Bob started playing Little League baseball when he was six. He had a good time but in the early days he wasn't very good. In his first game, a ball was hit to him and before Bob could catch it, it bounced and hit him in the nose. Grandpa yelled from the sidelines, "Use your glove next time." Again Bob missed Grandpa's humor just like he missed the ball.

When Bob was eight years old his baseball team got a new coach. George was very strict and told the players if they missed three practices, they were off the team. He was a good coach and the kids learned a lot. Bob had more opportunities than I did when I was young because George carefully followed the Little League rule, requiring everyone to play at least two innings.

Even though Bob was small and light, by the time he reached high school, he went out for the football team. When the senior players laughed, the coach told them at least Bob was trying out for the team.

Ryan was another freshman who, unlike Bob, did not try out for the team. Any physical talents Ryan might have had were devoted to being a bully. Ryan liked to pick on Bob because he wouldn't fight back. After a few weeks of this, Bob decided he wanted to learn karate in order to defend himself.

One day in P. E. class Ryan ran full speed and jumped in the air and faked a swing at Bob's face. When Bob brought his arm up in defensive karate move underneath Ryan's arms, he knocked him off balance. He fell and hit his head on the floor, got up and yelled to the teacher that Bob had knocked him down. The teacher saw this happen and for a long time had witnessed Ryan's bullying. When the teacher told Ryan he got what he deserved, the problem ended.

Bob was a member of Kaleidoscope, a song and dance group at the high school and their schedule conflicted with football, so he had to choose between the two. When we discussed this, Bob said he wanted to stay with Kaleidoscope because he was able to participate more. In football he practiced as hard as everyone else but didn't get to play much. He told me he went out for football to make me proud of him. I told him I would be proud of him no matter what he decided.

High School was tough for Bob but he always made the grade. After he graduated Bob went to DeVry Institute of Technology. Before completing his course work, he came home, got a job, and transferred to Lincoln Land Community College. He worked hard and went on to study computer science at the University of Illinois at Springfield, where he graduated with honors.

I've always admired his determination and am proud that he earned a degree in his chosen field. Still his most outstanding characteristic is his kindness and gentleness. Bob's always happy to help others. He has been a tremendous blessing to our family and an inspiration to me. From a young age Bob always looked out for me. Both he and Mary had seen the results when my back was bumped and my temporary paralysis frightened them. If I was in a position where someone could get behind me, Bob would move to protect me.

49

I had worked at the YMCA for about five months when my supervisor became ill and unable to work. The YMCA director didn't want Bill to feel any pressure and wanted him to know his job was secure until he was able to return. Bill often came to visit old friends and told me many times he was pleased with how well I was doing.

Finally, the doctors told Bill he wouldn't be able give massages any longer. I was told Bill wouldn't be back and when I asked for Bill's job, the YMCA director told me they wanted someone with more experience. He asked me to stay on until the new man was hired and I agreed. When I met the new health club director, I discovered he was a good masseur and we got along very well.

Illa and I were still having a difficult time paying our bills. My factory job and both our part-time jobs didn't meet our expenses. To pursue my career goal of being a masseur, I checked at the Elmhurst YMCA for jobs at other locations. I was told someone would look into the possibility and let me know. About a week later I received a call about an opening and after being told I would have to relocate, an interview appointment was scheduled for the following week in Chicago.

The two men who conducted the prescreening were pleased with me and I was offered a second interview at the work location in Springfield, Illinois. Illa and I discussed the move and prayed for the Lord's guidance. After a couple of days, we felt we had the Lord's blessing and we were at peace with the decision to move.

With Bob entrusted to Illa's parents, Mary joined us for the trip to Springfield. The two-hundred-mile journey gave us plenty of time to sound out our ideas.

When we arrived at the Springfield YMCA, we were given a tour of the facility which ended at the health club. Bill Masseke, the health club director introduced me as a possible masseur and one of the members said to me, "Let's see just how good you really are. I want you to give me a massage." I looked at Bill to gauge his reaction. He smiled and nodded his approval.

The man was in great condition, about six-feet tall and well over two hundred pounds. Being stiff from the ride to Springfield, this was just what I needed to loosen up. It was probably the best massage I had ever given and he was really impressed. He talked about how good my pressure was and how relaxed he felt. He could not get over how strong the massage was from someone not even five-feet tall.

After the massage he said, "Well, let's go."

"Where are we going?" I asked.

"It's time for the interview." We hardly sat down when he said to the members of the interview committee, "We need to hire this young man. He not only has tremendous strength in his arms, but he gives a great massage and has a great touch. We better not let him get away or we'll lose a great masseur."

The decision was made to hire me and I agreed to start in two weeks. When I returned to Springfield, Bill helped me find a room about two miles from the YMCA. The lady who rented the room couldn't do enough for me. She made my stay very enjoyable until Illa and our children could join me.

50

While our West Chicago house was on the market, Illa would make weekend Springfield visits to see me and look at homes. My boss referred me to a health club member, named Al in Sherman who built and sold houses. The next time Al came to the health club he told me about a good tri-level home across the street from his house. It was listed at a very good price and he offered to show it to me.

When I told Illa about the tri-level, her father decided to come to Springfield to see the house. He was very angry about our move and complained to Illa all during the trip. Illa called me during a meal stop to warn me about her father's mood and how nothing she said pleased him.

As soon as he walked into the YMCA, his anger shifted from Illa to me. He didn't want his daughter and grandchildren moving away from the family and I was the cause of the separation. I tried to explain that my reasons were financial and not personal. Even though I felt our relationship had reached a new low, I feared it was about to get much worse.

Arriving in Sherman to look at the home, we found it structurally sound, but it had water on the basement floor. My father-in-law's anger was close to the surface and he told the owner the water problem would need to be fixed.

On our way back to the YMCA, Illa asked her father what he thought of the house.

"There is a lot of work to be done on that house." Looking at me he said, "You can't fix anything. You didn't do a thing with the home in West Chicago and you won't do anything here either."

"You told me yourself that you didn't want me doing anything to the house. You bought it for your daughter and said that you would be making the repairs. If I wanted to do anything I'd have to have your permission. This house will be fixed up by me and I will do what has to be done. You might as well get used to the idea of us moving to Sherman, because we are moving. It really doesn't matter to me what you think."

After we stopped screaming at each other he said, "You know you owe me an apology."

"You're not going to get one from me."

"I ought to take you outside and give you the beating you deserve."

"Don't ask me to go out there with you because I'm just angry enough to do it. There will only be one of us coming back, and it won't be you." I didn't like to answer this way, but I'd had enough of him and I wasn't going to let him push me around.

I would never settle an argument with my fists, especially with my father-in-law. I always thought someday we could work through our bad feelings and fighting would only make this more difficult.

When I came home to West Chicago the following weekend, my father-in-law renewed his demand for an apology.

"After all you said to me, you think I'm the one who owes you an apology? Forget it. You're not getting one. I did not have the right to yell at you, but you had it coming. Everything I said still stands. That's the way it is, whether you like it or not."

Our offer on the Sherman tri-level, contingent on the sale of our West Chicago home was accepted. It seemed like a long time, but finally we were offered cash for our house. Illa called and said Dad felt we should take the offer. I told her I agreed and we took it. We moved into our new home on June 11, 1969. It took us a few weeks to decide how to arrange the furniture, but when it was finished, we were pleased by how nice the home looked.

51

In 1969, before the all–city swimming meet, a swimmer came into the health club with a sore shoulder. Joe was the star of his high school swim team and he had trouble lifting his right arm. My massage worked the spasm out and he went on to win all of his races. During follow-up massages, he told me about his football team and suggested I contact the coach.

I called Springfield High School and spoke to Coach Sowinski. I told him I'd just moved to Sherman and had worked on Joe who thought the football team could use me as a trainer.

He was very nice on the phone but said, "Our school can't afford to pay you for your services."

"I'm interested in helping your football team and willing to volunteer my services."

He seemed pleased and after thanking me for my offer asked about my experience.

"I've been working on injured athletes from Wheaton College for about ten years."

"How do you work on their injuries?"

"I start out by placing hot packs on the pulled muscles to stimulate circulation. Then I massage the muscles above and below the injury with analgesic oil."

I was a different type of trainer. Most trainers used stretching and rotation and never used massage as part of their treatment.

The coach must have liked what he heard because he invited me to the game that Friday night. "You can come, meet everybody, and just watch the game."

I went up to the gym early and Coach Sowinski introduced me to the players and other coaches. It was a hot, muggy night and during the game, the dehydrated players started having cramps. I went from player to player, massaging the athletes for the rest of the night. After the game the coach told me how pleased he was with how hard I worked and the following week I became the team trainer.

During one of the subsequent games a player was injured and the coach sent him to my home for a massage after practice on Monday. Tom complained of sore shoulders and trouble lifting his right arm. I ran my fingers over his back and shoulders, where I found muscle spasms, but no indication of an injury. Pressing gently down his arm to his elbow, I discovered a soft area that moved when I touched it. As soon as this happened, I knew I shouldn't give him a massage. God blessed me with very sensitive fingers and the wisdom to know when not to use them.

I went to the phone and called Coach Sowinski. "I think Tom has a blood clot in his arm, and should see a doctor right now. I may be wrong, but this could be serious."

"How did you know this was a blood clot?" the doctor asked after he removed it.

"My trainer felt it and thought I needed to see a doctor."

"You're very fortunate that your trainer found the blood clot. If you had played, a blow to your arm could have been dangerous."

"We have a great trainer," Tom told the doctor, "He's the best there is."

I was flattered when Tom told me about this, but I reminded him that God deserved the credit. My massage ministry had entered a new phase in a new location. I prayed to God every day for the energy to reach everyone who came to me. My interest was not money; it was serving people who were hurting and sharing God's love while giving the treatment.

52

While working at the YMCA, Bill taught me how to work on pressure points, showing me different approaches to relieve pain. He was a great mentor who always worked hard with me and we got along fine for the first year.

It was widely known that Bill was insecure and short-tempered, so some of the YMCA members often teased him. If Bill asked if they wanted a massage, they would say they would have me give them one because I was better than he was. Bill hated to be teased and became angry with their comments.

"Why do you listen to them?" I would say. "I know I'll never be as good as you. You have so much more knowledge and experience."

At first Bill listened to what I said, but over time our relationship deteriorated. His anger made it impossible for me to work with him. Once I took Bob to the emergency room and called the Y to leave a message for Bill that I would be late. The secretary didn't give Bill the message until he was ready to go to lunch. Since my absence prevented him from leaving, Bill exploded when I arrived an hour late. I was told the YMCA came first and if my children needed to see a doctor, my wife would have to take them. I couldn't do anything right for him, so I decided to look for another job.

Later that day a YMCA member, who was the Assistant Superintendent of Public Instruction for the state, came in for a massage. We had become good friends during the year I had been working on him and he questioned me about my mood that evening. I explained my problem with Bill and he invited me to see him in his office the next day.

When we met he told me about an opening in the accounting department and asked if I was interested. I was so surprised and happy to replace my problem with Bill with a promotion to a new job. I went back to the YMCA and gave them my two-week notice.

53

In 1971 I met Paul Jenkins, the new Williamsville High School football coach. I was introduced to Paul as a trainer and while he was very pleasant, he said he wasn't interested in having a trainer for his team. Coach Jenkins believed an injured player should play through his injury unless it was a major problem. This would teach him not to be controlled by pain and make him a better player.

I respected his point of view. I grew up with "old school" coaches who felt that way. Springfield High was the only school in the area that had a trainer, so the value of this service was not widely understood.

During the next few years, I worked my day job with the state and continued my volunteer work as a trainer for Springfield High. Athletes from many other schools came to our home for treatment. Even with longstanding school rivalries, sportsmanship prevailed when they joked around with each other. The few exceptions were dealt with swiftly and they followed my house rule of showing respect for each other. My free nights were always filled and through my massages God worked to heal many injured players.

With my daughter and son in the Williamsville School District, many of my neighbors urged me to leave Springfield High and work in my own community. I told them I was introduced to Coach Jenkins years before and at the time he wasn't interested, but I agreed to talk to him again.

Since my first meeting with the coach, some of his players had been coming to me for massages. They were able to return to the field following their injuries sooner than Coach Jenkins expected. Because of this my reception was much warmer than before. I left Springfield High and went to Williamsville as their trainer in 1977.

An hour before our Saturday games I would make sure all the players were warmed up with a gentle massage with a large vibrating pad. This relaxed the tension and made them more focused. When the energized team roared out of the locker room, all I had to do was stay out of their way.

When the weather was very hot, I used an ice towel to wipe the players' faces as they came off the field to prevent heat strokes. Due to my small stature, the players knelt in front of me so I could reach them. All such activities were secondary to my primary duty of caring for injuries.

Early in the season, our team captain developed a muscle spasm in his hips and asked if I could do something to take away the pain. As I applied the analgesic to Tony's hips, Coach Jenkins yelled for Tony to get back in the game. He jumped when the coach yelled and started to run back on the field with my hand stuck under his hip pad.

Tony stopped and turned toward me and said, "That's okay, Mr. Byron. I have to go back into the game." He started to run again toward the field with me attached.

"Tony," I yelled, "my hand's stuck." He stopped and as I pulled my hand out, I noticed the biggest smile on his face. Walking back to the bench, I heard the laughter of fans on the sideline.

Not all situations were this amusing. A few games later, one of our defensive linebackers tackled a running back so hard that he jammed his head into the runner's stomach. The impact stunned our player, leaving him motionless on the ground.

I rushed onto the field and reached under his shoulder pads and felt the tightness in his neck and back. I massaged it very gently until the paramedics arrived. I told them Mark had a muscle spasm and after a few minutes he began to move his arms. I was relieved to see this and thankful that God was watching over me.

The paramedics took Mark to the hospital and after the game I went to see how he was doing. To my surprise Mark was sitting up talking to the doctor. They had given him a heat treatment which released most of the severe muscle spasm and were keeping him overnight for observation.

Mark's example always inspired his teammates and I knew he would be returning to the team soon. I was impressed with Mark's desire and the tough spirit God had given him. He was going to play football and nothing was going to stop him. Following his release from the hospital, Mark saw me daily for massage treatments he was back on the field for the next game.

This was a great year for me at Williamsville. My treatment of Mark's injury made a strong impression on the team and my reputation as a trainer grew with time.

54

After four years in the accounting department at my state job, I transferred to the special education section, where I embossed and bound Braille textbooks. In 1979 I had just finished a book, walked over to put it on the shelf and turned to go back to the Braille machine when I fell. Unable to move my legs, I yelled for help. Coworkers ran in to help me and someone called for an ambulance.

During my examination at the hospital, we discussed my spina bifida and history of falls. After a couple of hours, movement returned to my legs and I was referred to my family doctor and released.

My neighbor, Dr. Olysav was doing an orthopedic internship at the hospital and asked his boss, Dr. Stauffer to examine me.

"You have a serious problem here," Dr. Stauffer said, looking at my x-rays. "A vertebra is sliding over another one and you need to have surgery. With the recovery period, it will take a year before you'll be able to return to work. I want you to go home and talk it over with your wife before you make a decision."

Later that evening Dr. Olysav came to our house and reviewed the options Dr. Stauffer had explained to me. Without surgery my life expectancy was three to five years. I'd have at least five and maybe ten years with surgery. My heart was strong, but this was a new and difficult procedure and there was a strong possibility I might not survive the surgery.

Dr. Olysav gave us the confidence to proceed with the operation. He was going to be in the operating room with me and this made both of us feel better about going through with it.

We felt this was the best choice and called Dr. Stauffer's office for a surgical appointment. We told him we wanted the surgery and he scheduled it for June 29, 1979. Dr. Stauffer said a second operation would be needed and he scheduled that one for the second week in July. With this decision made and the prospect of relief from pain, I felt more at peace than I had in years.

Dr. Olysav came to see me in the hospital the night before my surgery. We had talked many times leading up to this moment and I always found his concern and support very helpful.

"Jim, you're not afraid of this surgery, are you?" he asked.

"No, I feel whatever happens will be the Lord's will."

Illa and I looked forward to the possibility of relief from my severe pain and a longer life. While we were well aware the operation could cause my death, we turned our fears over to God and He provided peace in our hearts.

"You know, I talked to Illa," he said, "and she feels the same way you do. I just want you to know how very serious this is going to be."

"I feel safe knowing you will be there in the operating room. I know you will do everything you can to help me. I am in good hands because God will be there with you. Think of what I have before me, if the doctors are successful, I'll have a longer life with less pain and I believe that will happen. If I don't survive the operation, I'll be with God. So you see, I have the best of both worlds. It is a winning situation, regardless of the outcome."

"I admire your faith. I just pray God will choose to extend your life."

"Two other members of our church face serious surgery tomorrow and there is a special prayer meeting this evening. I'm sure they feel as blessed as I do. There will be so many prayers going to God that I feel that He will answer them and we'll be all right."

"Well, I'll be watching over you very carefully."

"I can't ask for more than that."

Dr. Olysav is a very special doctor who could see the Lord working in our lives. He was part of the reason I was not afraid.

The Lord watched over my six-hour operation and the doctors were very pleased with their success. On my way to the recovery room, one of my attending doctors reminded me they would have to do a second surgery. I didn't know what I was saying and told him, "Doc, I'm not doing anything this afternoon. Why don't you do it then, and we'll have it out of the way." He just laughed and said that I had to get over the first one before doing the second.

Following my recovery, the nurses brought me back to my room. I was uncomfortable lying on my back, but the doctors had told the nurses not to turn me over until 5:00 P.M. Each time a nurse came in, I'd ask, "Is it five yet?" When Dr. Olysav came in, he told me I'd just have to live with the pain for a few hours until it was safe to move me.

Finally, at five o'clock, a couple of nurses came in; one nurse held my hands and pulled me toward her. The other nurse was standing behind me gently supporting my back to help the nurse in front. The pain was intense. I yelled so loud it was a wonder that the other patients didn't stampede out of the hospital.

After that, the nurses came in every half-hour to turn me. It was good to move and even though the pain was still intense, it gradually diminished. By the fourth day I was able to move from side to side with very little pain.

Dr. Stauffer came to my room every day to check on my progress. The first surgery straightened my back and arrested the curvature problem that, over time, would have impeded the functioning of my heart and lungs. Two weeks after the surgery, he explained that the second operation would involve going through my stomach to reinforce what had been done during the first surgery.

Illa called Reverend Ken Cox and told him what the doctor had said. He came right to the hospital to see me. "Jim, keep your eyes on the Lord. He'll take care of you. If a second operation is needed, you must have it. Continue to look to Him and allow His spirit to guide you." Reverend Ken's love and support comforted me and helped me maintain a positive attitude. There was a second special prayer meeting at our church the night before my second surgery for me and other church members who needed the Lord's help.

The second surgery was done on July 12, 1979. Long steel rods were placed to reinforce my back. The surgery was very painful, but in about ten days the pain was gone.

A couple of days after my surgery, a nurse came into my room to wash my legs and feet. When she spread my toes, I said, "Hey that hurts."

"I'm sorry, Jim. I didn't mean to hurt you."

"That's okay. I couldn't feel anyone touching my toes before. This is the first time I felt you washing them."

"You be sure you tell your doctor. He'll want to know."

Later when I finally remembered to tell the doctor, he was very surprised and pleased with this new development. "That's a bonus for us," he told me.

I had been in the hospital for a long time and now it was time to go home. When we pulled into our driveway, the neighborhood turned out in force to welcome me. I was amazed and delighted by their response. There was impending rain and amid the occasional sprinkles everyone one greeted me on my return.

My new home for the next eight months would be our kitchen. Since I would be confined to a bed the entire time, the frequent activity of the kitchen would help me pass the time and I would be conveniently situated for meals. If I had been set up in our bedroom, looking at the walls and the limited view from a smaller window, it would have driven me crazy.

Illa purchased a used hospital bed that nicely fit the space. I was in a heavy body cast which covered my torso and was connected to my right leg to the knee. My range of motion was greatly restricted, but I was able to rotate my body from side to side. Looking out at the trees from my right side, I could admire the Lord's gift to the world. Turning to my left, I could see one of God's greatest gifts to me, my wife Illa and how nice she had made the kitchen look for me.

Illa's parents offered to help her take care of me for the next three weeks. We appreciated their thoughtfulness and willingness to take time out of their busy schedule. During their visit, a student came to see me.

"Mr. Byron, what is your favorite pie?" Lynn asked.

"Chocolate, banana cream, apple," I said. "I like them all."

"I'm going to make you a pie. I don't know how to cook, but I'll have a pie for you."

She brought the pie in on Sunday, kissing me on the cheek as she handed it to me. "Mr. Byron, you're always there for all of us. I just wanted you to know how much we love you."

This was just the beginning of an outpouring of love from the local school communities I had served over the years. Families brought in groceries or baked goods to make sure we had enough to eat. Our monthly house payments as well as gas and electricity were paid each month and we never knew who to thank. My in-laws sat back in silent witness to these acts of kindness to someone they had always felt was an unworthy son-in-law.

During the first week of their visit, the contentious relationship with my father-in-law continued as it always had. Even when he assisted me, he was rough and often caused me pain. From this point forward a change occurred. Perhaps seeing how other people regarded me caused my father-in-law's transformation. Now when he gave me a bath I experienced a gentleness I hadn't seen before. In an expression of sincere Christian love, he became like a servant answering all my needs.

I had a small bell and would ring it whenever I needed help. My father-in-law always responded kindly. When I sat on the bedpan, he took care of everything. I realized that he was doing this out love for me.

"You know Dad, you don't have to do this," I said. "I really appreciate how hard you are working to make me feel better."

"I know that you're going to have a tough time," he said, "and I just want to help." He said this with such gentleness that I knew his attitude had finally changed and I realized for the first time how fortunate I was to have him as a father-in-law. The anger we had felt toward each other was replaced with kindness and consideration and we became the best of friends that very moment. God's love changed our lives.

Six months after the surgery, Dr. Olysav wanted me up and walking. My goal was to walk around the bed two or three times a day to develop strength in my legs.

Before I could walk, I had to be able to stand. Standing took a tremendous amount of energy and it caused severe pain. After eight months in bed, reaching a standing position required slow incremental movements. At every step of the way, I'd have muscle spasms that caused me to fall back on the bed.

Once I was able to remain in a standing position, it was time to take my first steps. My ankles swelled and hurt in the beginning, but with exercise the pain gradually subsided and I was able to walk farther and farther.

Standing and walking were major accomplishments. For the first time in my life I was free of back pain and I couldn't believe the difference. My surgery was an astonishing success. This thrilling and tremendous gift from God was the answer to my prayer.

55

Over time my strength increased and I was able to walk longer distances. On a return visit my father-in-law was surprised by my progress and we decided to go shopping to look for new pillows. As we were leaving the store with our purchases, a driver failed to yield to pedestrians and almost hit me.

"Why didn't you hit him with the pillow?" my father-in-law asked.

"That would really put a dent in his fender, wouldn't it," I said.

We walked away laughing. Our relationship was becoming more like father and son, finally after all these years. This was the beginning of some great times together. We saw different sides of each other and liked what we saw. Anger and fighting were replaced with smart remarks that caused us to laugh at ourselves.

My increased energy level was rejuvenating and my children had a difficult time keeping up with my childlike exuberance. Whether we went shopping or to a movie, my children were worn out by the time we returned home. I'd fought so hard all my life to walk and now it was easy and something to enjoy.

By the following winter, I had the strength to shovel snow. I didn't dread this task; I felt the Lord blessed me with a new ability. What I didn't realize was a more incredible gift was yet to come.

In 1982, three years after my surgery, I received a letter from my mother-in-law. During her daily devotions she had reflected upon her daughter's twenty-year marriage to me, our past conflicts and difficult times. Her guilt was very heavy on her mind and she felt God lead her to ask for my forgiveness.

I read the letter over and over in disbelief. This was an unexpected development and when I shared it with Illa; she was as surprised and confused as I was.

I thought about how to respond for a long time. When I finally wrote to her, I said I had always tried to understand her point of view. As a parent I understood that we all want the best for our children and there had been times when I too did not feel worthy of having Illa for my wife.

I knew that once again God had opened a door for me and I wanted my mother-in-law to know how I yearned to have a good relationship with her. Since my own mother passed away she was the only mother I had. Regardless of her feelings toward me, I had always tried to love her.

From this point forward, our relationship began to change. We looked for the good in each other and enjoyed what we saw. The ability to appreciate each other was a blessing from God and made us feel better about ourselves. My mother-in-law became very considerate and whenever she called, her first question was, "How is Jim doing?" This newfound concern gave us a good feeling.

Each year my family went to Pittsburgh to spend time with my brother Tug and his family. During our weekly visits, Tug was always excited and animated. One year, soon after we arrived, I noticed he was uncharacteristically quiet. He had something on his mind and I wasn't sure what it was. After a couple of days, he said, "Jim, come with me." The force of his command made me follow in silence.

We walked down over the hill. Tug worked hard mowing and clearing the ground until their ten acres looked like a park. Finally, under a huge tree, Tug stopped and said, "I have something to tell you."

"What's on your mind?" I asked.

"I wish I could be like you. I've been thinking about you for a long time and wanted you to know how I feel. You endure so much pain yet never complain. I can see the pain in your eyes and the deep lines in your face. The pain never goes away does it?"

"No, it's always there," I said.

"You've spoiled me. People who work for me take time off when they think they're too sick to work. You'd work your shift without complaining. Nothing ever seems to bother you. No matter what happens, you can deal with it. I've often wondered how you handle things so well. You're an inspiration to me."

I'd never known anyone to look at me and feel as strongly as he did. I was really impressed with our very special relationship.

"Tug, you're the one I look up to. Whenever I face a tough situation, I ask myself, how you would handle it."

Tug had a tremendous influence on me and I wouldn't do anything to lose his respect or disappoint him.

During this time, my massage ministry continued to grow. Athletes from ten area high schools came to my home for treatment. There was always a full house and when it was Tammy's turn, she and her mother entered the treatment room. Tammy had missed a couple of games because of her painful injury and I could tell her spirit was very low. After the massage Tammy sat up. I touched her shoulder and told her she was very special, that God loved her and I did too. As she sat on the bench with her back toward me, I hugged her for a few seconds to allow the Lord to touch her heart.

Her mother was very pleased with my treatment and brought Tammy back the next week for another one. When I finished, I told Tammy she could get up off the table when she was ready and I turned to speak to her mother. Tammy said, "Mr. Byron. You didn't finish your treatment."

"Yes, I did," I said. "I did everything that needed to be done."

"No, you didn't. You forgot my hug."

When I realized how important this was to her, I gladly complied.

Two weeks later I was one of the adult leaders for a youth group lock in at our church. From 8:00 P.M. until 8:00 A.M., we played games, had prayer meetings and ate pizza. One of the kids suggested a new game.

"First, we choose someone we admire," Cherrilyn said, "and write down things we like about the person. Then we tell the one we chose three of the things."

After she passed out pencils and slips of paper, everyone began writing. When they finished Cherrilyn said, "I'll start. I'm picking Jim Byron, because he is always there for me, easy to talk to, and nice to us." I smiled and Cherrilyn approached me and gave me a hug. The young people had so much fun with this new game that it was all they wanted to do.

Cherrilyn classmates loved her and her Christian witness touched many hearts. She is an outstanding young lady who has been an inspiration to me and her gesture really impressed me. So many athletes at the Sports Therapy Center were feeling depressed by not being able to participate in their sport. Hugging was an expression of God's love that lifted their spirits and it became a standard practice after my massages.

56

Auburn High School had a good football team and it was always a hard fought contest whenever we played them. Williamsville's game in the fall of '84 was no exception. Auburn was ahead during the whole game and, with less than a minute to play, Williamsville had to score a touchdown to win.

Williamsville called a time out to decide what play to call to make the eight yards needed for a first down. It was fourth down and Williamsville was on its own 45-yard line, so the next play would decide the game.

Williamsville faked a hand-off up the middle of the line. The Auburn team went for the fake and tackled the guy they thought had the ball. Our halfback ran deep and was wide open. He caught the quarterback's pass on the 8-yard line and ran it in for the touchdown.

Our bench went crazy and I was as excited as everyone else. Standing next to me on the sideline was our assistant coach, Gerry Timm who was a foot and a half taller and outweighed me by a hundred pounds. He picked me up and swung me over his head and I felt something snap. As soon as he put me down, my ribs started to hurt. Coach Timm went to the other end of the bench to direct the defensive line. Suddenly I became dizzy and passed out on the playing field.

The Williamsville fans saw I was hurt and yelled at the coaches to alert them that I was lying on the field. The head coach finally saw me and called the referees to stop the game. Paramedics revived me, moved me off the field, and placed ice on my ribs and neck.

I came to the game with my minister and when he saw I was injured, he rushed to my side. The paramedics told me to be sure to go to the hospital. Reverend Ken said, "Jim has no choice. I'm driving and we will stop at the hospital."

Coach Timm was sorry he hurt me and was so upset that he kept calling my house until I arrived home from the hospital. I thanked him for calling and told him what the doctors had said.

Six mounts later my bruised and cracked ribs finally healed. The coaches continued to tell me to stay away from Gerry when we scored a touchdown. My ribs may have healed, but Gerry's ribbing went on for a long time.

By the fall of '86 the Williamsville football team had the highest team spirit I had seen in the nine years I had been their trainer. Growing up together and playing football since junior high, they could anticipate their teammates' moves on the field. Off the field they could tell when someone was troubled and they cared enough to want to solve the problems. Anyone could see the love and respect these young men showed each other.

While watching a professional game on TV, I saw one of the teams kneel down for prayer before the kickoff and I was reminded of the pre-game prayers at Wheaton College. I had always included the team in my prayers and I thought it might be time to include the team with my prayers. Things were always hectic before a game and other high schools didn't take the time to pray. Before each of our games, I could see our desire and dedication. This precious spirit touched my heart and I asked our coach if I could share a thought and a prayer before our games and he agreed.

Coach had the players form a semi-circle around me as I talked with them. It took just a few minutes and the young people were hungry for what God had to say. God used this opportunity to plant the seed of love and I was pleased that He allowed me to be a part of it.

"You must have your thoughts only on the responsibilities of your position to make the team successful. You must give your all for the team's benefit. During tough times, it's important for each one of us to lean on God and reach down into our hearts and pull out His energy and be focused to play to the best of our ability. It's important for the captains to look over at the bench after each play to see what defense the coach is sending in. If you don't look over, you are not doing your job and the team will suffer. If you make a mistake, don't hang your head, go back and look at why the mistake was made so it won't happen again.

"Always remember that you are special and I love you. But there is one who loves you even more than I do and He died on the cross because He loved you so much. His name is Jesus Christ. Now let's have a word of prayer."

57

I received a letter inviting me to the Bellwood Grade School reunion to be held at Crooked Creek State Park in Pennsylvania. The reunion included everyone who attended during the thirties and forties. Tug was the chairman of the reunion committee and asked all his brothers to attend. My wife and kids were looking forward to meeting all the characters I'd been talking about for many years. From my descriptions of the people in my hometown of McGrann and the many funny incidents that happened while I was growing up, my kids knew the people as well as I did.

Still the memories of rejection and the bitterness in my heart were ever-present. This was my problem and I had to handle it the best way I could. Illa knew how I felt and could tell I was apprehensive. She told me not to worry--people would be happy to see me. Having my three brothers at the reunion bolstered my courage and in the end we decided to attend.

When we finally arrived at the reunion, I stepped out of the car but hesitated before going over to join the party.

"Are you coming?" Illa asked. She stopped and waited for me to catch up.

"Give me a few minutes. I'll be right over." Illa went on ahead and sat down at a picnic table to watch how the people would greet me and see my reaction. Before me were the friends and enemies of my childhood. As eager as I was to see some of them, others evoked painful memories that I would carry with me forever. I took a deep breath and walked over to confront my past. If I encountered any put-downs, I planned to walk away. No one could have felt as low as I did at that moment.

There must have been two dozen people who recognized me and walked over to talk to me. Some knew about my recent surgery and were surprised I lived through it. They were so happy to see me and their hearts were filled with so much love. I couldn't believe what was happening. It was all that I could do to hold back my tears of joy.

Many told me how much they missed me and my being at the reunion made their day. The love that flowed from their hearts and into mine left no doubt that Christ had brought me to this reunion to heal me.

Standing among this diverse group--those who were nice to me and those who were cruel--shaking hands and hugging each other, I felt all the resentment that had built up for so many years dissolve and wash away. WOW! What a blessing.

58

Coach Butkovich, affectionately known as Coach B., was the Mt. Pulaski Basketball Coach, who like other coaches around the district brought their injured athletes to the Sports Center for me to work on. One night, in early November 1988, Coach B. waited until I had finished with everyone and said, "Jim, I want to talk to you. Please sit down."

I sat down and with a look of surprise said, "What's on your mind?"

"I'm nominating you to the Illinois Basketball Coaches Association Hall Of Fame as a Friend of Basketball."

"Why me?" I asked. "I haven't done any more than lots of other people."

"You've done so much for our area's high school basketball players that you've earned this."

"I can't believe it, but thank you."

"If the committee approves your nomination, you will receive an induction letter and two tickets to the dinner ceremony."

This was a beautiful surprise and a great honor. Coach B.'s thoughtful comments gave my spirit a lift.

The Williamsville High School principal called and asked for newspaper articles about my work as their trainer and about the Sports Therapy Center. I provided all of the information I had and he sent it on to the nomination committee.

Later that month I received a letter informing me that the Hall of Fame Committee had selected me for induction in April 1989. With the information packet, there was an application for the Hall Of Fame ring.

"It's great to be inducted into the Hall of Fame," I said, "but the ring's expensive and I don't need it to know that I've been inducted."

"Where is the application?"

"You don't need it, because we can't afford the ring."

"This is a special occasion," Illa said, "and I want you to have it. We'll find some way to pay for it."

A couple of months later Illa and I were invited to attend a Williamsville assembly, where I was asked to speak to the high school students. Whenever I had this opportunity, I told the students how very special they were to me. As I waited to deliver my remarks, a student took the stage to introduce me.

"As you all know, Mr. Byron will be inducted into the Illinois Basketball Coaches Hall Of Fame, which he truly deserves. We knew he was special long before his nomination and we are so proud of him." She turned and looked at me and said, "Mr. Byron, will you and your wife come up to the podium, please."

The crowd applauded as Illa and I joined her. "We have a surprise for you. Illa told us how much you wanted the Hall of Fame ring, so the students took up a collection to cover the cost of the ring and other expenses. On behalf of the students at Williamsville High School, it is my pleasure to present you with this check."

THE HEALING TOUCH 263

When it was my turn to speak, I was so touched that tears came to my eyes. "I came here today to share how very special you are to me. You know what you've done just shot down my little speech. That's okay because I feel your love could only come from Christ. I love you so much and I could never come close to saying what's in my heart. Thank you for this beautiful gift."

On the following Monday the ring came in the mail. When Dr. Meckes, the high school principal, saw me later he said, "You know Jim, no one loves you like our young people. Normally it takes a long time to raise money, but these students had the money for your ring in two days. That really says something to me about how special you are to our school."

I was also blessed by a gift from a group of sorority sisters who help fund activities at our local schools. They contribute to other causes and presented me with a check for my family's travel expenses to the induction ceremony.

The dinner was scheduled for April 29, 1989. This was a big week for me. Friends and family from Pennsylvania planned to join in the celebration. Tom Lasher, a friend I grew up with, called and said he was coming and he would have a surprise for me.

When my surprise stepped off the plane, I said to Illa, "That looks like my brother Dick."

Tom and Dick stayed at our house that night and we stayed up late reliving our past. Seeing Dick was a terrific surprise. The four of us met my brother Tug and his family at their hotel in Bloomington the following day. It was so nice see Tug and his wife, Betty as well as my nieces, Debby, Karen, Barby, and Debby's husband Chuck.

That evening at the Illinois State University Union Ballroom we enjoyed a wonderful dinner. While waiting for my time to go the podium, I prayed this ceremony would be very special.

My uncle Duncan Graham arrived late and came in as I was going up to receive my award. I walked up and stood next to Coach B., a man I greatly admired. As my accomplishments were read to the audience, my heart was pounding. Coach B. presented me with my plaque and gave me a hug. When I kissed him on the cheek, we received a standing ovation and I felt Christ's love fill the room.

Coming off the platform, I suddenly became light headed. I rejoined my family and I could tell by their expressions how very proud they were of me and my very special award. I sat down and thanked God for the blessing of this moment with my family. It was such a humbling experience, and yet the honor touched my heart.

My friend John Fanale made a video recording of the induction, which gave me the opportunity to relive this beautiful moment many times. Tom Lasher snapped many pictures of me going up to the podium. I would have enjoyed these pictures too if Tom had remembered to put film in his camera.

I received a letter from my Aunt Louise who wasn't able to attend the dinner. She wrote, "We all are very proud of you. You had the hardest road to travel and you never quit. All of your brothers are whole and you're the one with the disability that made you stronger, and you've gone farther than anyone had hoped you would. I can see your mother and father looking down from Heaven with big smiles on their faces because of how far you have come. What you have done is inspiring."

Aunt Louise's letter really touched my heart. I felt overwhelmed by her love. All my life I've wanted to make the kind of difference in the lives of others like my family had made in mine.

59

My father-in-law had been sick for about a year and by the time we gathered for Christmas, his condition had visibly worsened. Dad had lost weight and was weaker than when we saw him in August, so weak that he had trouble getting in and out chairs. When I asked if he needed help, he graciously accepted and reaching down to place my hands under his armpits, I lifted him very gently to make sure he didn't fall.

"I didn't realize how strong you were," he said.

"My strength is your strength. You're very special to me and I'm just glad to help."

One evening we decided to look at Christmas lights around the neighborhood. Walking to the car, Dad suddenly slipped and his feet flew out from under him. I had my arms under his armpits and lifted him off the ground so he wouldn't fall.

During this final visit with him, our children saw another side of their stern grandfather, the gentle loving side of a man who really loved his grandchildren. A couple of months after our beautiful time together, God finally called him home.

He was an outstanding Christian man, who visited men in jail to talk to them about Christ. He gave all he had all the time.

I really miss our spiritual relationship. He was not only my father-in-law, but a very dear friend who meant the world to me. I'll always remember the fun we had together and thank God for the privilege of knowing him.

When my mother-in-law read an early draft of my story, she relived the tough times I endured from the beginning of my marriage until my surgery in 1979. She apologized for the way she and her husband had treated me and noted how well we get along now.

Since she was presented in an unflattering light, I offered to take out or change those parts. She declined this offer because she felt others might benefit from our experience and reconciliation.

In the beginning, we had a lot of problems, but God stayed with both of us so that we could work them out. I learned a hard lesson--regardless of how badly we treat each other, with God's love to guide us, we can always reach a peaceful solution.

60

Sunday dinners at our house after church have been a long family tradition. In the fall of 1998, our five-year-old grandson, Dain, came into our bedroom and said, "Grandpa, can I talk to you?"

"Sure Dain, what's on your mind?"

"When you were very young, you almost died, didn't you?"

"Yes, that's true."

"When you were older, you almost died again, isn't that right?"

"You're right, I was very sick."

"When you were in the hospital, even though you were sick, you helped people get better. Grandpa, how can you help people when you're that sick? I know when I don't feel good I don't want to help anyone."

"Dain, God knows what's best for all of us. When high school students came to visit me, I was able to give them massages to relieve their pain. God made my concentration so strong that I forgot about my own problems."

"I wish I could do that. You know Grandpa, the kids in my class say I'm lucky to have someone as special as you."

"That's really nice, Dain."

"Do you know I've never heard anything bad about you?"

"No, I didn't know that," I answered.

"Do you know what I think?" he asked.

"No, tell me what you think."

"I think you're the greatest."

"That's really special, Dain."

"Someday when I grow up, I want to be just like you."

"You mean you want to be short like Grandpa?"

"No, I want people to love me the way everyone loves you. If I have that I'll have everything."

"Dain, do you realize what you've said?"

"Yes Grandpa, I want people to say nice things about me the way they do about you."

"Thank you, Dain."

"You know what else I think?"

"No, tell me."

"I think you're awesome." Dain kissed me on the cheek and walked out of the room.

I was impressed and humbled by how beautifully Dain expressed himself. My young grandson had reached a new level of spiritual love. Tears filled my eyes as I sat in my chair and felt God's spirit touch my heart.

Dain remains a blessing to me. Today our love for each other is stronger than ever. I will always remember that priceless time when the gentle words of a child blessed my spirit. For me Dain's love for others is a beautiful example of how to serve God. He continues to inspire me to witness to others and be the awesome grandpa he saw so long ago.

61

In 2008 the Williamsville football coaches established the annual Jim Byron Award presented to the player who best exemplifies the spiritual, athletic and academic values of the team.

In 2011 the Sangamon County Community Foundation established the Jim Byron Scholarship Fund which provides a $1,000 award to the most deserving Williamsville graduate.

As I look back at my life, these awards are especially gratifying because since my birth I was not expected to even survive let alone achieve anything. The fact that I had a wife, children, a grandchild and a career, as well as a spiritual ministry working with injured athletes from fifty schools defied all expectations. I owe it all to the support of my family throughout my life but most of all to our faith in God who has always been there for us. My life proves that with God's love anything is possible.

COMMUNITY FOUNDATION
for the Land of Lincoln

205 South Fifth Street
Suite 930
Springfield, IL 62701
Thanks to Bill Hahn who recommended Jim for the
Williamsville High School
Jim Byron Scholarship
Established 2011